Delavier's

Women's Strength Training Anatomy Workouts

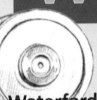

Frédéric Delavier

Michael Gundill

Human Kinetics

Library of Congress Cataloging-in-Publication Data

Delavier, Frédéric.
 Delavier's women's strength training anatomy workouts / Frédéric Delavier, Michael Gundill.
    pages cm
 Includes bibliographical references.
 1. Muscles--Anatomy. 2. Weight training for women. 3. Muscle strength. I. Gundill, Michael. II. Title.
 QM151.D4512 2014
 612.7'4082--dc23

                              2014021047

 ISBN: 978-1-4504-6603-5 (print)

This publication is written and published to provide accurate and authoritative information relevant to the subject matter presented. It is published and sold with the understanding that the author and publisher are not engaged in rendering legal, medical, or other professional services by reason of their authorship or publication of this work. If medical or other expert assistance is required, the services of a competent professional person should be sought.

Developmental Editor: Julie Marx Goodreau; **Associate Managing Editor:** Nicole Moore; **Copyeditor:** Patsy Fortney; **Senior Graphic Designer:** Nancy Rasmus; **Cover Designer:** Keith Blomberg; **Illustrations (cover and interior):** © Frédéric Delavier; **Photographs (interior):** © Human Kinetics; **Photographs (back cover):** Courtesy of Frédéric Delavier; **Photo Production Manager:** Jason Allen; **Art Manager:** Kelly Hendren; **Associate Art Manager:** Alan L. Wilborn; **Printer:** Versa Press

Human Kinetics books are available at special discounts for bulk purchase. Special editions or book excerpts can also be created to specification. For details, contact the Special Sales Manager at Human Kinetics.

Printed in the United States of America.   10 9 8 7 6 5 4 3

The paper in this book is certified under a sustainable forestry program.

Human Kinetics
Web site: www.HumanKinetics.com

United States: Human Kinetics
P.O. Box 5076
Champaign, IL 61825-5076
800-747-4457
e-mail: humank@hkusa.com

Canada: Human Kinetics
475 Devonshire Road, Unit 100
Windsor, ON N8Y 2L5
800-465-7301 (in Canada only)
e-mail: info@hkcanada.com

Europe: Human Kinetics
107 Bradford Road
Stanningley
Leeds LS28 6AT, United Kingdom
+44 (0)113 255 5665
e-mail: hk@hkeurope.com

Australia: Human Kinetics
57A Price Avenue
Lower Mitcham, South Australia 5062
08 8372 0999
e-mail: info@hkaustralia.com

New Zealand: Human Kinetics
P.O. Box 80
Mitcham Shopping Centre, South Australia 5062
0800 222 062
e-mail: info@hknewzealand.com

Delavier's
Women's Strength Training Anatomy Workouts

Contents

PART III Programs

Introduction

Every woman can benefit from strength training regardless of her age or goals. Younger women can use strength training to sculpt an attractive body they can keep all their lives. Athletes can increase their strength or endurance by training with weights.[1,2] Active women can benefit from being fitter, more attractive, and healthier at any age. Weight training helps all women cope with daily stress, fight obesity, and avoid cardiovascular problems. It is also the best tool for reshaping the body after giving birth.

Resistance training benefits middle-aged women by counteracting many of the health issues associated with menopause by preserving the integrity of both bones and muscles. It also mitigates the fat redistribution that can cause adipose enlargement in the abdominal area and result in plenty of loose skin in the arms.

Seniors can slow down aging by having stronger muscles and more resistant bones. Better muscular control and balance may preclude falls. Moreover, proper maintenance of range of motion can forestall a loss of mobility.

Clearly, resistance training benefits go far beyond appearance. This healthy habit can help us all live longer and better. Health, after all, is not just a gift from heaven. Although genetic predisposition plays an important role, medical research shows that genetics accounts for only 30 percent of health.[3] The other 70 percent is determined by lifestyle. In other words, we are responsible for our health.

Physical inactivity is associated with a significant decrease in life expectancy. For example, every hour spent being inactive results in a life expectancy loss of 21 minutes.[4] For a woman watching six hours of television per day, this translates to a decrease in life expectancy of almost five years.

Large-scale research studies have shown that sedentary people who exercise 15 minutes per day increase their life expectancy by three years compared to completely sedentary people.[5] To counteract the deleterious effects of inactivity, weight training and cardio training (e.g., running, cycling, aerobics) provide the greatest health benefits in the least amount of time.

Resistance exercise is designed to put extra pressure on the muscles; however, in the process, it places pressure on the tendons, ligaments, and joints as well. When resistance training is done properly, the added pressure results in a strengthening effect; however, done improperly, that pressure can damage tissues. Weight training should be a healthy habit, not a health hazard. Therefore, injury prevention is a major focus of this book. The goal of a fitness program is to build the body, not destroy it.

Part I provides a very simple, yet thorough explanation of how to tailor a training program to suit both your goals and your schedule. Part II describes in detail the best exercises for each region of the body. Complete training programs to get you started are outlined in part III.

Weight and cardio training will not only improve your appearance but will also improve your health and change your life for the better. It's time to get started.

PART I
Developing Your Training Program

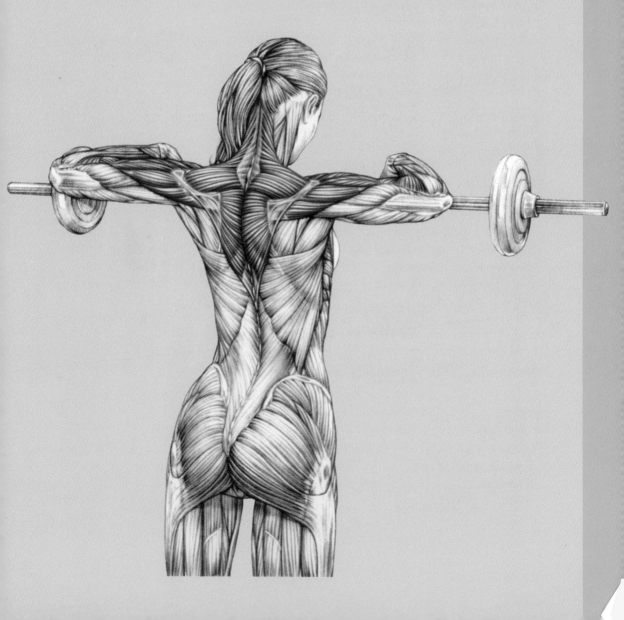

Developing a training strategy is the key to your progress and ultimate success. This is the first thing you need to do before setting foot in a gym or setting up a home exercise space; otherwise, you are going to get lost sorting through the varying pieces of advice that will bombard you.

20 Steps to Creating a Personalized Program

Creating your own program involves 20 steps, which are described in this section. They will give you the answers you need to start training with a program that best matches your goals.

The 20 steps outlined here combine resistance training and cardio training. You may have decided that you want to perform only resistance training. However, if you have fat to lose or have difficulty maintaining your body weight, it is wise to add some cardio training. Stretching regularly to maintain flexibility as well as good posture is also important, especially given that it requires only a few minutes per week.

Rigorously following a good program will result in progress. However, gauging progress can be difficult because you see yourself every day. You may even believe that you are not making any progress at all. And then one day your clothes feel tighter in a new place and looser in another. One way to detect improvements is to photograph yourself at least once a month. Many have found that photos are more reliable than body weight or measurements. Rest assured that as long as you are training regularly and eating a balanced, healthy diet, fat will diminish and muscles will develop. Because some women achieve results more quickly than others, though, you cannot predict your rate of progress.

1. Identify Your Goals

To create a perfectly tailored weight training program that suits your needs, you must first clearly define your objectives. You work out to do one or a combination of the following:

- Reshape your body
- Get rid of excess body fat
- Improve your sport performance
- Remain healthy
- Fight the loss of mobility due to aging

You should be able to precisely state your main goals as they relate to these objectives. Avoid very vague objectives such as *I want to get in shape* or *I want to improve my physique.* Be as precise as possible. For example, in one month, you may want to do one or more of the following:

- Lose 10 pounds
- Increase your strength by 10 percent
- Fit into clothes you have not been able to wear for a while

Specific programs to help you meet your goals can be found in part III of this book. There you'll find programs and circuits using either minimal equipment you can keep at home or gym equipment to focus on your upper body, lower body, or both. Ideally, you should tailor these programs to suit your specific needs. The following steps will help you do just that.

2. Decide How Many Days Per Week to Train

Your personal schedule will determine how many days you can work out each week. The following two weight training programs are suited to beginners:

- **One weekly weight training session:** Training only once a week is better than no training at all, and you will still make progress. For athletic women who are already training for their sport, one weight training session per week is probably enough. If you are a beginner with very little free time, this is a good start as long as you stick to your program.
- **Two weekly weight training sessions:** Two weight training sessions per week is a good minimum. If you train for a sport, don't overdo it by weight training more than twice a week.

If you are not doing sport-specific training to start with, we recommend that you perform two weekly weight training workouts for a month or two, and then move to three sessions a week when you feel ready. After three to six months of regular three-days-a-week weight training, if your body has adapted well to the rigor of training, you could move to a four-day program.

- **Three weekly weight training sessions:** If you do not practice any other physical activity, the ideal would be to work up to three weight training sessions a week. With this schedule, you can spend more time on each body region. If you are a beginner, training three times per week allows you to set up three shorter workouts as compared to two longer ones; if you have a couple of months of training under your belt, this schedule allows you to perform more sets per body region.
- **Four weekly weight training sessions:** This schedule allows you to perform even more sets and more exercises per body region. This is an advanced strategy that is not for beginners, even if it is tempting in order to make progress more quickly.

We do not recommend more than four weight training workouts per week. Keep in mind that overtraining is more damaging to your progress than undertraining. Only high-level athletes benefit from more than four sessions per week.

Muscle strengthening occurs only if you take enough rest between workouts. Therefore, rest is of the utmost importance if you want to progress quickly. Training too often does not provide your body enough rest. A loss of strength is the main sign that you are overtraining—in other words, that you are doing too much.

Women suffer from a higher risk of injury during sports than men do. For example, in response to resistance exercises, the rate of tendon collagen synthesis is 50 percent less in women than in men.[1] As a result, tendon regeneration is much slower in women than in men. Therefore, to avoid injuries, women need longer rest periods between heavy lifting sessions than men do. Alternating heavy workouts with lighter ones favors recovery.

As far as cardio training is concerned, if you wish to gain muscle mass and strength, do not overdo cardio; once or twice per week is enough. If you already train for another sport, no extra cardio training is required. For health purposes, performing three cardio workouts a week is enough to begin with. If you are in a hurry to lose weight, you can start with three short cardio sessions per week. As your endurance increases, you can slowly increase either cardio frequency or duration, or both.

3. Choose Your Training Days

To progress quickly, follow this one main rule: One day of weight training has to be followed by at least one day of rest from weight training (so doing a cardio workout the day after a weight training session is a possibility). This may not always be possible, but this is the ideal frequency. For the various schedules, here are your options:

- **One weekly weight training session:** This schedule does not pose any recovery issues, and weight training can be done on any day.

- **Two weekly weight training sessions:** Separate workouts as much as possible (e.g., Monday and Thursday or Tuesday and Friday), but at a minimum, try to respect the pattern of one workout and one day of rest. If you can train only on weekends, however, go ahead. Weight training on both Saturday and Sunday isn't ideal, but your body will have plenty of time to recover during the rest of the week.

- **Three weekly weight training sessions:** With this schedule, respecting the one-workout-one-day-of-rest pattern is difficult, but still possible. The worst possible configuration would be to train three days in a row and then take four days of rest. Try to balance your week as much as possible—for example, by weight training on Monday, Wednesday, and Friday or on Tuesday, Thursday, and Saturday.

- **Four weekly weight training sessions:** With such a high training frequency, properly spacing the workouts to provide your body with enough rest is difficult. Respecting the one-workout-one-day-of-rest pattern is not possible for at least two workouts. Whenever you perform two workouts without rest between them, make sure that one targets your upper body and the other targets your lower body.

Cardio training has fewer constraints because it does not traumatize the body nearly as much as weight training does. However, it is still a good idea to spread out the sessions as much as possible over the week.

4. Decide Whether to Train More Than Once Per Day

We strongly advise not to weight train twice a day, although you may do a weight training and a cardio session in two separate workouts per day if you do not wish to do cardio right before or after weight training for weight loss purposes.

Ideally, cardio can be performed on days you do not weight train. But it is conceivable to do cardio in the morning and weight training later in the day. Alternatively, you can weight train in the morning and do cardio at night. However, it is far easier to do cardio and weight training at the same time. See the cardio section at the end of this part to learn about possible combinations of these two forms of training.

5. Choose Your Training Time

Is it better to train in the morning, at noon, in the afternoon, or in the evening? Scientific studies have shown that muscle strength and endurance vary throughout the day.[19] Most women are stronger in the afternoon and weaker in the morning. But for a minority, it is the opposite! It would be abnormal, however, to have a constant level of strength and stamina throughout the day.

These normal diurnal variations are explained by the increase in body temperature throughout the day. The body is a little bit colder in the morning, and it slowly warms up with time and as a result of eating. This slight elevation in temperature is associated with an increase in central nervous system efficiency. Therefore, muscle power rises in parallel with body temperature.

Training whenever your muscles are at their strongest is ideal. For most women, this peak performance occurs in the afternoon. Unfortunately, it is not always possible to train at that time. If you can train only in the morning, your body will get used to it and gradually reschedule its peak strength. The worst-case scenario is constantly changing your training schedule, because it gives your body little chance to adapt.

6. Choose an Order in Which to Work the Muscles in Each Session

Training your whole body in one workout would be cumbersome. This is why we divide the body into regions. Following are the six major body regions:

1. Legs (quadriceps, hamstrings, glutes, and calves)
2. Abdomen
3. Back
4. Chest
5. Arms (biceps and triceps)
6. Shoulders

The main issue is how to combine these body parts to train them in the most efficient manner. Because of the many possible sequences, beginners often have difficulty figuring out a proper combination. The following four tips can help you design your program. They are discussed in detail next.

1. Take full advantage of the indirect work.
2. Rate the importance of each muscle according to your goals.
3. Focus on your weak areas.
4. Use the rotation principle.

Take Full Advantage of the Indirect Work

Basic chest exercises such as presses recruit the triceps as well as the front part of the shoulders. Basic back exercises such as pull-downs and rowing recruit the

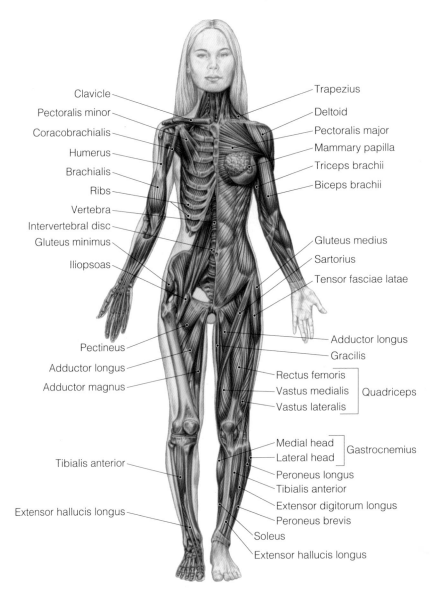

Clavicle
Pectoralis minor
Coracobrachialis
Humerus
Brachialis
Ribs
Vertebra
Intervertebral disc
Gluteus minimus
Iliopsoas

Trapezius
Deltoid
Pectoralis major
Mammary papilla
Triceps brachii
Biceps brachii

Gluteus medius
Sartorius
Tensor fasciae latae

Pectineus
Adductor longus
Adductor magnus

Adductor longus
Gracilis
Rectus femoris
Vastus medialis
Vastus lateralis

Quadriceps

Medial head
Lateral head

Gastrocnemius

Tibialis anterior

Peroneus longus
Tibialis anterior
Extensor digitorum longus
Peroneus brevis

Extensor hallucis longus

Soleus
Extensor hallucis longus

biceps as well as the rear part of the shoulders. Therefore, if you have performed these exercises, to save time, you can reduce the number of, or even skip, direct exercises for the arms as well as for the shoulders.

What you do not want to do is train your arms before your back or chest. This results in the biceps or triceps being too tired to handle the weight necessary to stimulate the chest and the back. Therefore, always train your arms at the end of your workout, or not at all.

The same goes for your legs. Training your calves first will tire them and decrease your strength for the basic leg exercises. Furthermore, the quadriceps and hamstring exercises provide enough indirect calf stimulation to render direct lower-leg exercises superfluous in many cases.

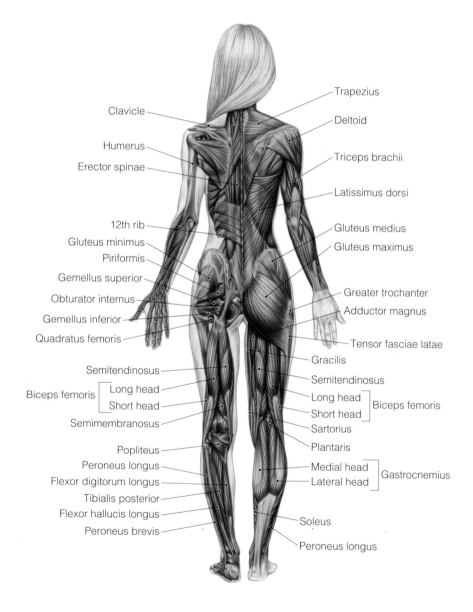

Trapezius

Clavicle

Deltoid

Humerus

Triceps brachii

Erector spinae

Latissimus dorsi

12th rib

Gluteus medius

Gluteus minimus

Gluteus maximus

Piriformis

Gemellus superior

Greater trochanter

Obturator internus

Adductor magnus

Gemellus inferior

Quadratus femoris

Tensor fasciae latae

Gracilis

Semitendinosus

Semitendinosus

Biceps femoris ⌈ Long head
          ⌊ Short head

Long head ⌉ Biceps femoris
Short head ⌋

Semimembranosus

Sartorius

Popliteus

Plantaris

Peroneus longus

Medial head ⌉ Gastrocnemius
Lateral head ⌋

Flexor digitorum longus

Tibialis posterior

Flexor hallucis longus

Peroneus brevis

Soleus

Peroneus longus

Rate the Importance of Each Muscle According to Your Goals

The glutes and the arms do not possess the same degree of importance for every-one. For example, women often tend to focus on their glutes and legs, whereas men concentrate on their arms. A woman who wants to focus on her glutes should spend far more time on her lower body than on her upper body.

Your program has to reflect your goals. If you want an aesthetically pleasing body, you should not treat all your muscles the same way. Many women prioritize the lower body and spend less time on the upper body. This is the most time effective combination to make quick aesthetic progress.

If you want chiseled abdominal muscles, you can begin each workout with abdominal exercises as a warm-up. If those muscles are not a priority, you can work them at the end of a session with whatever energy and time you have left.

Athletes must determine the degree of involvement of each of their muscles in their sports. For example, soccer players mostly train their legs and abdominal muscles and spend little time on their upper bodies. For volleyball players, the lower body is important, but the arms and shoulders are crucial, too. Therefore, they spend less time on the lower body and more on the upper body than soccer players do.

Focus on Your Weak Areas

Muscles don't progress at the same rate, and people are weaker and stronger in different areas. If your quadriceps strengthen or tone more easily than your hamstrings, it is important to train your hamstrings first, before your quadriceps. If you do not have any really weak muscles, you may want to apply the rotation principle instead.

Use the Rotation Principle

If you wish to develop a balanced physique, don't start each workout with the same body part. In the three-sessions-per-week example in step 7, one lower-body session starts with the quadriceps; the next one, with the hamstrings; and the last one, with the glutes.

When considering the previous information, be aware that there is a fundamental difference between training your muscles for aesthetics or health and training them to increase athletic performance. When training for sport, all the muscles should be worked on the same day, because in most sports, muscles work together and not individually. In that case, separating the muscle groups is counterproductive.

7. Schedule Your Body Regions for Each Workout

This step builds on step 6 to help you structure each workout. As noted earlier, your body is composed of six major body regions. The relative importance of each region is something you need to rank for yourself based on your aesthetic or performance goals.

If your goal is improved athletic performance, the demands of your chosen sport or activity will determine the relative importance of each body region. Do not give each body part the same degree of importance and therefore equal training time. Your specific goals should dictate your priorities and the training frequency each muscle receives.

If you want to make quick progress in strength and body shaping, the best thing to do is to work each muscle group twice a week. For losing weight, to maintain health, and for sports, working each muscle with weights only once a week is a good start. You may want to increase this frequency whenever you have more free time.

One Weekly Weight Training Workout

With only one weekly training session, you should spend most of your time on the lower body and abdominals and devote only a few sets to your back and shoulders. This way, the arms and the chest will be trained indirectly, which saves time. As you progress, you will have to add more sets and more exercises for each body part. This requires more training days to reduce the volume of work you have to perform during each workout.

Two Weekly Weight Training Workouts

As you increase the number of workouts, each muscle has more opportunities to be trained. In the examples for the two, three, and four weekly workouts provided here, the abdominals are included in the upper-body workouts, but the abs can be used as a variable and placed with the lower body in order to match the volume of work across the upper-body and lower-body workouts, which you'll see in the programs in part III. If you always train the abdominals with the upper body, the upper-body workouts could become too long and cumbersome.

Workout 1

Lower body: quadriceps and glutes

Upper body: abdomen and shoulders

Workout 2

Lower body: glutes and hamstrings

Upper body: abdomen and back

Three Weekly Weight Training Workouts

When you reach a point where your workouts are too cumbersome because you have to either perform too many sets or too many exercises to keep progressing, you can add a new weight training day to your schedule in order to lower the volume of work you have to perform for each workout.

Workout 1

Lower body: quadriceps and glutes

Upper body: abdomen and shoulders

Workout 2

Lower body: hamstrings and glutes

Upper body: abdomen and back

Workout 3

Lower body: glutes

Upper body: abdomen, chest, and arms

Four Weekly Weight Training Workouts

When you feel comfortable with your recovery while strength training three days per week, you can move to four weekly weight training workouts. However, this is an advanced approach that isn't appropriate for beginners.

Workout 1

Lower body: quadriceps, hamstrings, and glutes

Upper body: abdomen

Workout 2

Upper body: abdomen, shoulders, and back

Lower body: glutes

Workout 3

Lower body: glutes, hamstrings, and quadriceps

Upper body: abdomen

Workout 4

Upper body: abdomen, chest, and arms

Lower body: hamstrings

8. Determine How Many Exercises to do Per Body Region

As you will discover in part II, there are plenty of exercises for each muscle. Obviously, you cannot perform all of them in a single workout. It is neither possible nor desirable. You will also quickly find out that you like some of the movements and dislike others.

If you are new to weight training, it is wise to stick to a single exercise per major muscle: the one that you feel works your muscle the most (more about this crucial issue in step 18). After a couple of weeks, you can add another exercise for your major muscles (quadriceps, hamstrings, and glutes). It is best to stick to a single exercise for the less important body regions such as the arms and chest. For the more complex muscle groups such as the back, shoulders, and abdomen, you can decide whether to stick to the one-exercise rule or add another one depending on the importance you give to each body part.

After a couple months of training, you can add more exercises, but only to the body regions you wish to reshape the most.

9. Choose the Number of Sets Per Muscle Group

Once you have performed your exercise once, how many more times should you repeat it (i.e., how many sets of this movement should you perform)? The number of sets is critical because it is one of the major determinants of the duration of your workout. We all want to perform as many sets as possible, especially when we start training, to hasten our progress. Unfortunately, the body does not function well that way. There is only a finite amount of beating our muscles can handle without being overly exhausted. Past an optimal point, they will not be able to recover. Being overly tired and wishing to avoid another workout is an obvious sign that you have done too many sets.

For aesthetic purposes, muscles can artificially be divided into the following three major categories:

1. Most important muscles: quadriceps, hamstrings, and glutes
2. Complex muscles: back, shoulders, and abdominals
3. Less important muscles: chest, biceps, triceps, forearms, and calves

Beginners should aim for the following totals:

- Two or three sets for each of the most important muscles
- One or two sets for each of the complex muscles
- One set for each of the less important muscles

After a couple months of training, you should aim for the following:

- Three or four sets for each of the most important muscles
- Two or three sets for each of the complex muscles
- One or two sets for each of the less important muscles

After six months of training, you should aim for the following totals:

- Four or five sets for each of the most important muscles
- Three or four sets for each of the complex muscles
- One to three sets for each of the less important muscles

Keep in mind that the number of sets provided does not include the warm-up sets. You should be aware of your energy level before each workout. If one day you feel strong, you can perform more sets than usual. On the other hand, if you feel tired, do not hesitate to reduce the number of sets for that day.

10. Choose the Number of Repetitions Per Set

How many times (repetitions) should you perform an exercise in each set? For muscle toning, it is best to do from 10 to 20 repetitions with heavier weights. To burn calories and fat and to improve your cardiovascular health, do at least 30 repetitions, and up to 50, with lighter weights.

Determining the number of reps can be explained using a pyramid. This concept can be used whenever you perform more than one set per exercise. The pyramid system is used primarily with lower reps and heavier weights. When using lighter weights and higher reps, only increase the weight if you can remain within your targeted rep range; if you cannot, reduce the weight rather than the number of reps.

Here's an example using three sets. Once your muscles are fully warmed up (see how to specifically warm up each muscle group in part II), start with a light weight and a high number of repetitions (e.g., 20) for the first set. For the second set, increase the weight enough so that you can perform only 12 to 15 repetitions. However, do not stop during a set (except for the warm-up) because you have reached your repetition goal. If you were shooting for 12 reps but could do 16, go ahead and do them! For the third set, add weight so that you can perform only 10 repetitions.

11. Decide How Long Your Workout Should Last

How much time should you devote to each workout? This issue is very important not only to get fast results but also, and more important, to be able to stick to your program. You do not want to use too long a workout as an excuse not to go to the gym. A brief workout is much better than no workout at all.

Even minimal training provides muscle gains. One researcher has shown that, in women, as little as two minutes of daily resistance training for 10 weeks increased the rate of torque development by 16 percent.[3] Thus, it is wiser to train briefly but more often than for a very long time less frequently.

We believe that a 15-minute workout is better than a 2-minute workout. If you are a beginner, a 15- to 20-minute workout is ideal. After one to two months of training, try 20 to 30 minutes. After six months of training, 30 to 45 minutes should suffice.

The duration of your workout does not have to be fixed. If one day you have more time, do more sets or more exercises or target more body regions. If on another day you have less time, concentrate on the most important regions for your goals, or reduce your rest time between sets. A major mistake is believing that a good solution for skipping a workout is training twice as long during the next one. It is not. Regularity is crucial!

If you do not have time to go to the gym, there are plenty of exercises you can do at home with minimal or no equipment. In other words, do not skip workouts. This is of the utmost importance! If you skip one workout, you will skip another and then another. Next thing you know, you have not trained for months.

The objective of a good workout is to stimulate muscles to their maximum in the shortest time possible. What you should look for are strategies that increase a workout's intensity rather than its length.

The primary criterion that determines the duration of your workout is your schedule. If you do not have a lot of time, you can do a complete workout in a short time—for example, 10 minutes of circuit training (see the section Increasing Intensity). However, a 30-minute workout is still preferable.

A good weight training workout lasts at least 30 minutes and up to a maximum of 45 minutes. If you spend more than one hour working out, your effort is not intense enough. At the end of 30 to 45 minutes, your muscles should be begging for mercy.

The duration of your workout depends on two things:

1. Volume of work (number of exercises plus number of sets)
2. Rest time between sets

Rest time is the factor you need to adjust if you do not have enough time for your workout. Do not weight train for more than an hour because this means that you are doing one, or a combination, of the following:

- Working too many muscles per session
- Doing too many exercises
- Doing too many sets
- Taking too much rest time between sets

12. Learn the Proper Speed for Each Repetition

The speed of your repetitions is a very important factor in the success of your program. Do not lift a weight with too much speed by using momentum and body swings instead of your own muscle strength.

If you are just starting weight lifting, use a deliberate tempo rather than an explosive motion. You will quickly realize that a slower motion is more excruciating than a fast one. You use your muscles much more when you lift a weight up and down slowly, which is exactly what you want.

The key to rep speed is remaining in control of the weight rather than letting the weight control your motion. This is especially true at the beginning of a set. As your set progresses, you will start to lose control of your movement; however, this does not mean that you should stop trying to keep as much control as possible.

When you handle less weight using a deliberately slower speed, you will experience the following results:

- Your muscle fiber recruitment will be much more powerful.
- You will feel your muscle contract much more efficiently.
- You are less likely to damage your joints or tear a muscle.
- You are less prone to making a faulty move or losing your balance.

We recommend that you take two or three seconds to raise a weight and at least as much time, if not slightly more, to lower it. The weaker your muscles are or the older you are, the slower each repetition should be performed. The elderly are trained with much success using a super slow motion of 10 seconds to lift the weight and 10 seconds to lower it.[2] If this extremely slow motion seems too slow for you, raise the weight in five seconds and lower it in three to five seconds.

13. Determine How Long to Rest Between Sets

Consider your rest time between sets as a tool to help you reach your goal faster. If you mainly wish to sculpt your muscles, you need to rest long enough so that you recover most of your strength. On the other hand, you do not want to rest so much that your workout loses its intensity despite the heavier weight. If your goal is mainly to burn fat, do not rest much. Following are good between-set resting guidelines:

- To tone up, 30 to 45 seconds of rest should suffice. If you have no endurance because you just started weight training, you may want to rest more. But as you progress, you should shorten this rest time to respect the guidelines as much as possible and to ensure that you do not waste too much time in the gym.

- To burn calories and fat, you should adopt a faster pace with only 10 to 20 seconds of rest between sets. As you progress, reduce this resting time to a bare minimum. Once you have achieved that, you are ready to move on to the most intense form of weight training: circuits. Of course, with circuit training, your rest time between exercises should be limited to the time you spend moving from one exercise to the next.

Research has shown that women performing a similar workload as men produce less lactic acid and experience a lower elevation of heart rate. Therefore, they require less rest than men do between sets.[4]

Nevertheless, women tend to increase their rest period more than necessary to handle heavier weights and do more sets.[5] This decreases the intensity of a workout. Therefore, time yourself so that you stay within the time frame you set. This will keep you from resting too much.

14. Avoid Rest Time Between Two Different Exercises

Avoid wasting time when changing exercises. The time required to move from one machine to the next and adjust the seat or the weight (or both) provides enough rest. You might even have to wait for someone to finish a set. Do not add this compulsory wait time to a voluntary rest you just took. Moving fast burns both more calories and more fat while cutting down on the time you spend in the gym.

15. Pick the Proper Weight for Each Exercise

At first, choosing the proper resistance for each exercise may seem complicated. It doesn't need to be. Start with a resistance that seems too light to be challenging for your muscles. This easy set will serve as a first warm-up.

For the next warm-up set, increase the resistance slightly. If you hesitate, wondering whether the increase might be too much, pick up a weight that is too light and perform more repetitions rather than use too much resistance with sloppy form.

For your real first working set, increase the resistance even more, but again, not too much. If the weight feels too light during the first repetition, interrupt your set and pick up a more appropriate weight. By the same token, if the movement feels too difficult, stop your set and reduce the resistance.

For your second working set, you might increase the resistance slightly more to render the movement more challenging. But if your muscles feel tired, stay with the same resistance or reduce it slightly.

There is no fixed rule, here! You have to remain flexible regarding the amount of resistance. Whenever you perform more repetitions than expected, pick up a slightly heavier weight for the next set. Whenever you perform fewer repetitions than expected, pick up a slightly lighter weight for the next set.

It is very helpful to note each of your weights as well as the number of repetitions you performed for each exercise in a notebook or in your phone. There are plenty of apps for this.

16. Know When to Increase Resistance

If you scrupulously note all your workouts as suggested, you will easily figure out when to increase your weight for your next workout. If you do not write down your weight, you will face a very tedious task.

As a rule of thumb:

- If you performed more repetitions than expected for an exercise in your last workout, pick up a slightly heavier weight today.
- If you perform fewer repetitions than expected for an exercise in your last workout, use the same amount of resistance until you feel very comfortable with that weight.

You will not always be correct in your decision to increase your training load. Do not worry; nobody can predict future performances with 100 percent accuracy. However, you will be correct far more often if you have written records of your past performances than you will be if you rely on your memory.

Warning: If you had a very good workout last time, on paper, you may believe that you are ready to handle heavier weights. However, keep in mind that a very good workout takes a greater toll on the muscles and therefore on the recovery processes than an average training session. Therefore, your muscles may not have fully recovered and, as such, may not be ready to handle heavier weights. By the same token, recovering from a mediocre workout is easier than recovering from a standard workout. This is why most bad training sessions are followed by an increase of strength. Take this into account in your decision to modify your resistance.

17. Choose Exercises That Suit Your Morphology

Because of the variety of movements, starting a training program can be confusing. You have to realize that not all those exercises will suit your needs, and even fewer will suit your body biomechanics.

Everybody's morphology is unique in terms of height and the length of torso, legs, and arms. Some exercises force us to adopt unnatural positions, whereas others feel very natural to us.

If a movement places you in an uncomfortable position, eliminate it from your routine. When you start lifting, stick to movements that you feel your build is designed to perform safely. As a rule of thumb, the taller you are, the more dangerous the basic free weight exercises will be because you have to go through a much greater range of motion. This is typically true of the squat and the chest press.

By the same token, body weight exercises such as push-ups are likely to be more traumatic for your joints, also because of this greater range of motion. Part II identifies movements for which safety depends greatly on body biomechanics.

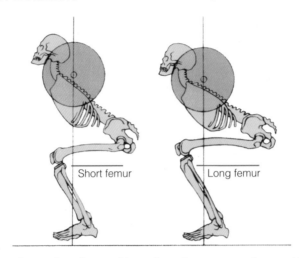

Short femur   Long femur

▌ Short femur, less forward lean; long femur, more forward lean

Machines Versus Free Weights

The two main kinds of resistance in weight training are free weights (dumbbells and bar) and machines. You may wonder which is more effective. As you will discover in part II, some muscles, such as the hamstrings, are difficult to train without machines. On the other hand, free weights are more appropriate for body parts such as the biceps. For this reason, a combination of both is best. It is a common belief in the gym that free weights are more effective than machines. This is simply not true. The most effective way to make progress is to use machines whenever they are more appropriate than free weights, and free weights whenever they are more appropriate than machines.

We are very much in favor of machines for beginners because they are typically much easier to master and better guide your movement as you learn the exercise. In addition, many new machines provide quick response (QR) codes that allow you to view a video of how to use the machine on your smartphone. You do not have to rely on anyone to demonstrate the proper use of the equipment. Of course, there is no such QR code on free weights.

Many studies point out that, for beginners, strength gains occur more rapidly with machines than with free weights.[6-8] This is because little motor learning is involved with machines because the movement is completely guided; this prevents errors of trajectory and balance issues. This very limited learning curve makes machines more appropriate for beginners. Women starting weight lifting are more likely to make better progress with machines than with free weights. During a 12-week study in which sedentary women followed a weight training program, one group trained exclusively with machines and the other with free weights. Muscular strength increased twice as much in the women who trained on machines.[7]

As you progress, you can move on to more complex, free weight exercises. They will be easier then because your muscles will have gotten used to the workout.

Starting directly with free weight movement is more complicated because it involves motor learning that will slow down your gains of muscle strength.

Two Major Exercise Subcategories

All movements, be they with body weight, free weights, or machines, can be divided into two major categories: basic, multiple-joint exercises and isolated, single-joint exercises.

1. **Basic, multiple-joint exercises:** Whenever more than one joint is flexed, the exercise is classified as a basic, multiple-joint exercise. For example, in a leg lunge, the knees, ankles, and hips are mobilized. Basic movements are more demanding than isolated movements, and they save time in your workout by working multiple muscles, but they are more complex to master.

2. **Isolated, single-joint exercises:** Whenever only one joint is flexed, the exercise is classified as an isolated, single-joint exercise. For example, in the leg extension, only the knees are mobilized. Because of the lesser demand on the body, isolated movements are easier to perform than basic, multiple-joint ones. However, because they recruit fewer muscles groups, they are less effective in terms of strength gains and calorie expenditure.

If your athletic abilities are minimal, use mostly isolated movements to rapidly improve your mind–muscle connection. After a few weeks of such training, you can progress to more basic exercises.

All movements, whether basic or isolated, are easier to perform on machines than with free weights. Keep this in mind if you have no athletic background because you do not want your new training program to be too hard on your muscles and joints.

18. Recognize When It's Time to Change Your Program

If you are new to weight training, we suggest you maintain the same training program for as long as you are making gains on it. It is counterproductive for beginners to frequently alter their routines because of the motor learning process required to assimilate new exercises.

Once you are familiar with weight training, feel free to change your exercises as frequently as you wish because there are few learning curves as you introduce new movements.

19. Take a Break

After a couple months of weight training, you may wonder whether to keep on training nonstop or to take a short break. If you go on a vacation or feel as though you need a break, it is fine to stop training for one or two weeks. But remember that when you stop working out, you do not burn as many calories; if you do not watch your diet, you might accumulate fat easily.

20. Maintain Your Gains

By the same token, you may wonder whether you should continue to intensify your training or to taper it when you are satisfied with your strength gains. The good news is that maintaining muscle gain is easier than acquiring it. However, researchers have shown that the volume of training required to maintain gains varies with age. People between 20 and 35 years old who have trained three times a week can maintain all their gains with a single weekly workout. Unfortunately, elderly people who have used the same protocol need two weekly workouts to maintain their strength.

The data for athletes who weight train during the off-season are similar.[20] They can maintain their strength level with a single weekly workout. On the other hand, one workout every two weeks is not enough for maintenance.

Increases in muscle strength occur well before muscle toning. The augmentation of strength can be very rapid because all the fibers within a muscle learn how to contract together, something that they don't do very well in sedentary women. Second, all your muscles learn how to properly coordinate their efforts, again something they are not good at in untrained women. With these increases in muscular efficiency, strength and endurance will improve first. Then, as a result of the manipulation of heavier poundage, hypertrophy, and thus toning, slowly occurs.

If strength increases rapidly as you first start training, its reduction occurs quickly if you stop working out for a while. Muscle shape is more resistant to a long rest period, which demonstrates that the reduction of strength is mainly due to a temporary weakening of the nervous signals. Your peak strength will return to its maximum within a couple weeks of training.

Increasing Intensity

Many techniques are available to increase the intensity of your training. The most obvious are adding weight and increasing the number of repetitions. These techniques use the overload principle. Both are excellent ways to put more stress on the muscles, but they also place more tension on the joints and ligaments. You should use them because they are the basis of resistance training; however, other techniques increase the level of training intensity without traumatizing your joints so much. These nontraumatic techniques are described in this section.

Muscle Burn

As your set progresses, your muscles feel as if they are burning. As you perform more and more repetitions, the intensity of this burn amplifies. This painful sensation is caused by the accumulation of waste known as lactic acid that gets trapped in the working muscles.

The muscle burn pain is a signal that you are pushing your muscles past what they are accustomed to. As a result, they have to become stronger and more resistant, which also translates into increased muscle definition.

Because it makes you uncomfortable, lactic acid may seem like an enemy. One goal of weight training is to turn this obstacle around and transform it into an opportunity for progression. Your main concern should be to learn how to generate and tolerate as much muscle burn as possible. Trying to achieve more muscle burn is a good alternative to handling heavier weight because it is safer on the joints.

Continuous Tension

Maintaining continuous tension in the muscle throughout the repetitions is a good way to increase difficulty without increasing weight. This requires that you not relax your muscles at any time during the exercise.

As you know, most weight training exercises have a top portion and a bottom portion, during which the muscles have a moment to rest. At the top of an incline press, for instance, when the arms are fully extended, the skeleton supports the load, relieving the tension on the muscles for a brief moment before the weight is lowered.

To maintain continuous tension, you must avoid the completely extended portion of the exercise by keeping your arms or legs slightly bent (contracted) at all times. This causes an intense muscle burn because of intracellular asphyxiation that occurs as a result of blocked circulation. Without oxygen, the muscles produce a lot of waste (lactic acid) while synthesizing energy.

Here is how to apply the principle to various exercises:

- During back, biceps, and hamstring movements, do not straighten your arms or your legs completely in the *stretched* position.
- During chest, shoulders, triceps, and quadriceps exercises, do not straighten your arms or your legs completely in the *contracted* position.

Note: Except for the deadlift, there is no loss of tension at the top of the contraction phase in back and hamstring movements. This differs from most of the basic chest and quadriceps exercises, in which tension is often lost at the top of the contracting phase.

Descending Sets

Using descending sets allows you to continue a set once you have reached fatigue without having to cheat. It involves briefly stopping the movement to rapidly remove around one third of the weight you are using and immediately resume your set. This allows you to continue the exercise and keep the muscle burn going.

For example, imagine that you are performing some barbell curls with 30 pounds (13.6 kg). At failure, you remove 10 pounds (4.5 kg) and resume the curls for a few extra reps. If you wish to push your muscles extra hard, whenever you reach failure again, strip down another 10 pounds (4.5 kg) and immediately start the exercise again. In general, you should not lighten the weights more than twice during a single set.

Supersets

A superset involves moving from one exercise to the next without taking any rest between movements. This technique allows you to work even more beyond failure than you can using descending sets. The two main forms are antagonistic supersets and supersets for the same muscles.

Antagonistic Supersets

Antagonistic supersets consist of doing an exercise for one muscle followed immediately by another exercise for the antagonistic muscle. For example, you start with a quadriceps exercise such as the leg extension and follow it with a hamstring exercise such as the leg curl. The goal here is to save time by not having to rest between sets. The muscles of the quadriceps recover while you train the hamstrings, and vice versa. Following are the main antagonistic supersets:

- Crunch for the abs and hyperextension for the lower back
- Incline press for the chest and machine pull-down for the back
- Lateral raise for the shoulders and rowing for the back
- Biceps curl and pulley triceps extension

With antagonistic supersets, by moving quickly from one exercise to another, you shape your muscles while increasing their endurance and burning more calories and fat.

Supersets for the Same Muscle

A superset for the same muscle consists of doing an exercise for a muscle followed immediately by another exercise for the same muscle. The goal is to increase the time under tension and muscle burn. If you use less weight for the second exercise as compared to the first, this superset also acts as a descending set.

You can choose your exercises for this type of superset based on one of the following rules:

1. **Postexhaustion exercises:** Start with a basic, multiple-joint exercise. When you reach exhaustion, move on to an isolating exercise. For example, for the buttocks, use maximum weights for the squat. At exhaustion, move to a hip extension machine such as the Butt Blaster. The squats alone may not induce an intense muscle burn in the glutes, but by moving to the Butt Blaster, your glutes will soon be on fire.

2. **Preexhaustion exercises:** Start with an isolating exercise. When you reach exhaustion, move on to a basic, multiple-joint exercise. For example, start training your buttocks with a machine such as the Butt Blaster. At failure, go directly to the squat or the lunge. By the time you perform your second exercise, your whole legs—not just your buttocks—will be on fire.

Circuit Training

An artificial separation of muscle workouts characterizes classic weight training. After several sets of an exercise for the legs, for example, you move on to exercises for the back. However, this is not the way the body works. In real life and in most sports, all the muscles work together.

Circuit training differs from classic weight training in that you perform a single set for a muscle group and then move on to a set for another muscle group, and then another until you are back at the beginning again to repeat the circuit, without resting. This develops endurance and burns more calories and fat than regular training.

If you dislike cardio or don't have time to do weight training plus cardio, circuits are the way to go. The cardio element is built in by virtue of the lack of rest between sets, and workouts are shorter, for the same reason. Because you can do shorter workouts, circuit training is a great time-saver. Part III provides circuit training examples.

Preventing Injuries

Your safety is our primary concern throughout this book. It should be for you, too! You do not engage in fitness to end up injured within a couple of months. Some types of workouts, such as CrossFit training, may look like a lot of fun, but they are also incredibly risky for your body. Researchers reported a 16 percent rate of injury during an intense CrossFit training program of 10 weeks.[9] This high injury rate occurred despite the fact that the program was closely supervised by well-trained professionals. Under the supervision of lesser-trained people or on your own, that rate would likely be higher. You are in fitness for the long term, to improve your appearance and your health, enhance your mobility, or slow down the aging process. Weight training should not deteriorate your health to the point of constant pain.

What about the milder forms of exercise such as yoga and stretching? The truth is that they are safer than weight training and cardio, but by themselves, they are not potent enough to significantly increase both muscle definition and muscle strength, or to preserve bone density. On the other hand, they are a great addition to resistance training!

Weight training can prevent spinal pain by increasing back muscle strength and improving posture. It is also a very effective way to reduce the level of pain of existing joint injuries.[10] But some exercises, even performed properly, can damage discs or joints. Therefore, it is important to point out the dangers inherent in each exercise and explain how faulty execution can increase the risk of injury. Part II exposes the most dangerous movements and provides the safest, most effective ones.

Women are more prone to injuries than men are because their joints are smaller and placed at more extreme angles and because of their hormonal fluctuations. As a result, not only are they more susceptible to joint injuries, but their injuries tend to be far more serious than the ones men sustain.[11]

Importance of the Warm-Up

You can sustain an injury even while performing a very safe exercise if you do not warm up sufficiently. This is especially true as you get stronger. As you begin to be able to handle heavier weights, the warm-up becomes more and more critical. When you are not very strong, the joints and the tendons do not need much warming up because the muscular tension required is not significant. As you gain strength, you will need to increase your warm-up time, because you will be subjecting your muscles to tension that more and more closely approaches their point of rupture. Part II provides complete warm-up routines to properly prepare your body before training any muscle group.

Importance of Head Position

The position of your head has a profound impact on muscle contraction. When you lean your head back, the lumbar muscles supporting the spine contract reflexively while the abdominal muscles have a tendency to relax. Even if the contraction is not very intense, these responses are inevitable. When you tilt your head forward, the abdominal muscles contract and the lumbar muscles relax. As a result, the body has a tendency to arch forward. This is why when you are standing up and looking up, you tend to fall backward. When you look down, you tend to fall forward.

You must have a clear strategy for the position of your head during weight training exercises. By all means, avoid moving your head from side to side. These unhelpful movements interfere with muscle contraction and could cause problems in the cervical spine. Except in unilateral exercises, never turn your head to the side. And if the exercise requires that your head be turned to the side, never move it during the exercise. In the same way, it is totally counterproductive to shake your head vigorously when the exercise gets really hard. Whenever your body needs to work hard, it is of the utmost importance to avoid any unnecessary head movement.

During abdominal exercises, keep your head tilted forward, and, above all, do not look at the ceiling. When you squat, keeping your head high helps your balance and protects your spine. If you move the head from left to right, the small reflex contractions that follow will alternatively recruit and then relax the muscles on the left side and then the right. This will interfere with the proper execution of the exercise.

Training-Induced Headache

A training-induced headache is not, strictly speaking, an injury, but it is nonetheless a health discomfort related to physical exercise. Therefore, it is an issue that should be addressed because it tends to affect women more than men.

The training-induced headache was first described by Hippocrates in 450 BC. Fortunately, it affects only a minority of women. As they start training, a mild to serious headache develops. This pain can last from a few minutes to a day and prevent them from training altogether.

If you suffer from this condition, you should warm up very slowly and thoroughly to prevent it or at least postpone it. Avoid increasing the intensity immediately. Perform a few minutes of easy cardio to get your blood moving. Despite what is usually recommended, start your workout with a smaller body part and a light isolating exercise such as the shoulder lateral raise. Use compound movements such as squats or deadlifts at the very end of your workout because they are the most likely to trigger a headache if you are prone to it.

Stretching

Over the years, strength training can reduce your range of motion by tightening your muscles. A certain amount of muscle and tendon tightness is necessary, especially in strength sports, but too much inflexibility combined with a restricted range of motion can result in injuries.

However, flexibility is not an end in itself. It can be impressive, but being too flexible works against performance. This is because very flexible tendons and muscles render the joints less stable and thus more prone to damage and injuries. Women's tendons are already much more flexible than men's are. This is one reason their joints are looser and more prone to injuries. If your joints are already unstable, stay away from stretching the muscles surrounding them. This is very common at the shoulder level. Strength training can tighten the shoulder joints so that they become more stable and less prone to injuries. However, don't avoid all stretching exercises just because you have an unstable shoulder. You can still stretch your hips, your lower back, your ankles, and other areas.

Joint Laxity During Menstruation

The risk of injury, especially of ligaments, is much greater in women than in men. For example, the incidence of tearing the cruciate ligaments of the knee is three times higher in female athletes than in their male counterparts. This vulnerability is largely due to a higher secretion of estrogen in women than in men. It is especially true during the preovulatory period.

By the same token, hormonal fluctuations during this period cause increased flexibility in the muscles and tendons, suddenly rendering the joints less stable. The resulting joint laxity can cause false movements. Birth control pills mitigate

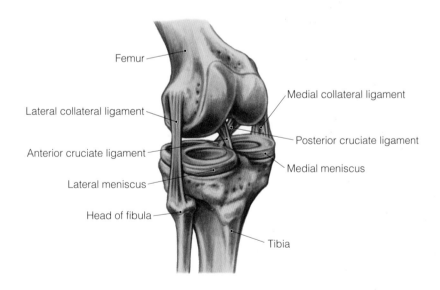

Femur

Medial collateral ligament

Lateral collateral ligament

Posterior cruciate ligament

Anterior cruciate ligament

Medial meniscus

Lateral meniscus

Head of fibula

Tibia

the natural hormonal fluctuations and tend to reduce the incidence of injuries due to joint instability.

Whenever you notice a sudden increase in joint laxity, stop stretching that joint. Also, reduce the amount of weight you are using on the exercises that mobilize that joint because the risk of injury has skyrocketed. Wait for stability to return to normal before resuming heavy training and stretching.

When to Stretch

Following are four good times to stretch your muscles. You do not have to stretch at all four of these times: Choose the approach that suits you best, which for many people is after each workout.

1. **During the warm-up:** Pretraining stretching may improve performance, but most often, it is likely to reduce muscle strength if performed excessively. Like stretching a rubber band, when you stretch your muscles for a few seconds, they, and their related tendons, heat up. However, stretch them too far and, like a rubber band, they lose strength and could even snap.

   Research shows that warm-ups with sustained stretching are generally associated with reduced strength.[21] Losing even a small amount of reactivity causes a muscle to be less explosive, because the stretch–shortening cycle is slower. This reduced performance lasts only a few hours, but it is enough to reduce strength during your workout. So be careful not to overdo it when you stretch as part of your warm-up. Always stretch a cold muscle gently.

2. **Between sets:** Stretching during your workout can have two consequences: (1) It allows you to rapidly regain muscle strength, which helps reduce the resting time between sets, or (2) it accentuates a loss of strength. There are explanations for both reactions that depend primarily on the amount of muscle fatigue achieved during the set. With that in mind, stretching could be beneficial between the first few sets of a workout when you are stronger and counterproductive during the later sets, or vice versa. You will feel the benefits or drawbacks of stretching right away. Pay attention to what your body is telling you; do not be rigid about stretching between sets. Even if some people praise the virtues of stretching, the benefits do not apply for everyone all the time.

3. **After the workout:** Following a workout is the best time to stretch because a temporary reduction in muscle strength, if it occurs, will not be an issue. Ideally, you should stretch the muscles you have just worked because they will be warm. But keep in mind that being too flexible can harm your long-term performance by destabilizing your joints. Your goal is to achieve a good range of motion so you can maintain good posture and prevent injuries.

4. **Between workouts:** Stretching can be used to speed recovery between workouts. However, contrary to popular belief, stretching between workouts does not always help muscle recovery. The problem with this strategy is that you start with cold muscles, which can be dangerous.

How to Stretch

There are three stretching techniques to consider: static, ballistic, and dynamic.

1. **Static stretching:** Static stretching consists of holding the stretch position for 10 to 30 seconds. The degree of stretch has to be modulated according to your level of flexibility. If you are not flexible, do not stretch too much or for too long. As your flexibility improves, you can intensify the degree of stretching.

2. **Ballistic stretching:** Ballistic stretching combines small bursts of stretching with small recoils of muscle contractions. You can repeat this combination of small, back and forth movements for 10 to 30 seconds. We do not recommend this form of stretching to beginners; it is a dangerous technique that allows you to stretch beyond your natural flexibility.

3. **Dynamic stretching:** Dynamic stretching uses movement, often sport-specific movement, to achieve a stretch. It is different from static stretching in that an end position isn't held; it is different from ballistic stretching in that there is no bouncing motion that can force the stretch beyond your natural flexibility. Walking lunges, arm circles, and leg swings are examples of this type of stretch.

Cardio Training

Weight training and cardio (aerobic) training are two very different forms of exercise. Yet, they are very complementary. Medical researchers have shown that cardio training favors fat loss, whereas resistance training enhances lean muscle mass as well as strength.[12] Cardio tends to reduce lean body mass, whereas resistance training is 30 percent less effective than cardio in shedding fat.[12]

Furthermore, aerobic activity is most appropriate for improving endurance and cardiovascular health. Therefore, it is better to combine the two types of training rather than to practice only one.

Breakdown of Cardio Versus Weight Training

The respective importance you should give to each form of training depends on your goals. Consider the following:

- If your priority is to lose body fat, you should mainly perform cardio training. However, do not neglect resistance training to preserve your lean mass. It is best to spend two thirds of your time performing cardio exercises and only one third performing weight training.

- If you mainly want to tone your body, devote two thirds of your time to weights and one third to cardio.

- If you desire to tone up and lose fat at the same time, divide your training time equally between weights and cardio.

- If you are too skinny, you can skip cardio as you attempt to gain as much muscle as possible.

Cardio Training Methods

The two most popular types of cardio are cycling and running, whether on machines or outdoors. What is the most effective way to burn fat? Researchers compared the energy expenditure of athletes while they were either running or cycling. In both cases, the intensity (60 percent of $\dot{V}O_2$max) and exercise duration (120 minutes) were similar. [22]

The use of carbohydrate as fuel was relatively similar: A gram of sugar per minute was burned in both cases. However, the researchers concluded that running burns more fat than cycling, which is exactly what you want to lose weight.

In summary, running may be more beneficial than cycling to lose weight. However, running is much more traumatic for the knees, hips, and lower back.

The treadmill is obviously less traumatic than classic running. Biomechanical studies have shown that to reduce the pressure on the knees and the hips, it is best to use slower, long strides rather than short, fast ones. A stair stepper is a great alternative to running, especially because it targets the glutes more than the treadmill does.

If you suffer from joint pain, use common sense and opt for the less dangerous form of cardio—cycling—even if it is somewhat less effective. To compensate, just ride longer or with a little more intensity.

Keeping a Workout Notebook

It is important to keep a workout notebook so you can easily recall the number of repetitions you did for each exercise as well as the weight, or resistance, you used. Note the duration of your workouts as well. Time measurement is important because, if you rest longer between sets, your performance will improve, but it will not necessarily result in strength gains. To compare two workouts, you must ensure that they are of approximately the same duration.

After each workout, examine your training session and ask yourself the following questions:

- What worked well?
- What did not work well?
- Why did it not work well?
- How can I improve my next workout?

How can you determine whether you really used the proper form in each exercise? An easy way is to film yourself. If possible, do so from a different angle at each successive set. It can be very surprising to see yourself train because the fluidity of the movement is not always what you imagine. Using this feedback, you can immediately self-correct and thereby improve your form. High-level athletes frequently use this strategy to enhance their techniques.

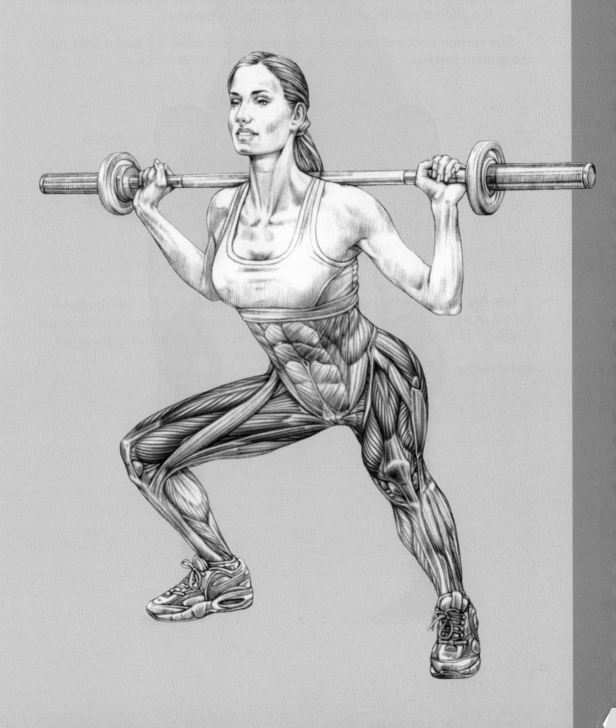

PART II
Exercises

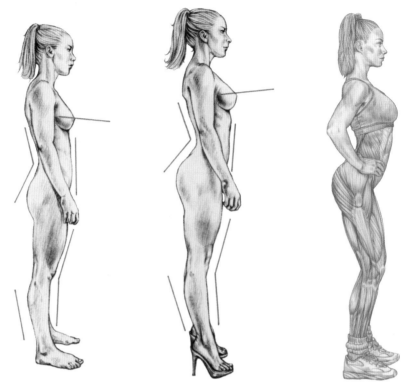

▌ **Wearing high heels will alter your posture, rendering your silhouette more attractive. Weight training can mirror these alterations, without the high heels.**

To visualize what you are trying to achieve, consider a woman's overall posture and appearance while wearing high heels; specifically, the lower back is slightly arched and the glutes are more visible. By weight training your glutes properly, you can achieve the same effect without the high heels.

Take-Home Lesson for Women

There are plenty of body weight exercises for toning the glutes. They work wonders at first, but their main limitation is the lack of resistance they provide. After a while, as your muscles get stronger, these exercises become too easy. You may perform more and more repetitions, but this is not the best way to get fast results. You have to overload the glutes with constantly heavier weights to get them to respond.

Because at first any repetition pattern provides results, it is best to remain below the 25-repetition range for toning. To achieve that goal, you have to add extra loads to your legs. By adding ankle cuff weights, you can easily overload your glutes. Unfortunately, in general, ankle cuffs weigh only 10 to 20 pounds (around 5 to 10 kg). They will help you for a while, but this is far from enough weight to challenge the glutes over a long period of time as you get stronger.

Besides ankle weights, you can use ankle straps that hook you up to a cable machine. This way, you can easily and gradually increase the amount of resistance. This issue of proper resistance is also the reason glute machines were created. The exercise these machines have you perform is not any better than the movement you can do with your own body weight. The difference is simply that machines allow you to easily add resistance to really overload the glutes, which is the key to rapid results in muscle toning.

Understanding Cellulite

Cellulite is a plague for many women. Development begins in adolescence, when girls start to release more and more female hormones. Both estrogen and progesterone favor the growth of fat cells, particularly in the lower body. This fat proliferation impairs the microcirculation of blood in the lower body, which triggers localized inflammation. As a result of this blood flow restriction and inflammation, extra water is retained in the legs and bundles of collagen that give the skin its firmness become damaged. This looser skin explains the orange peel appearance of cellulite.

Your genetic background also plays a major role in the localization of fat deposits around your glute area.

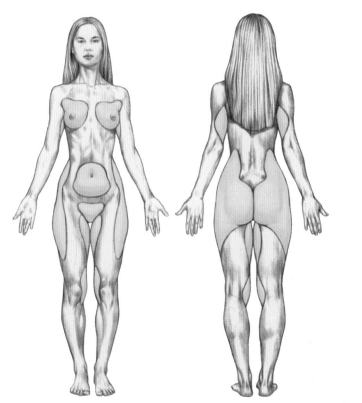

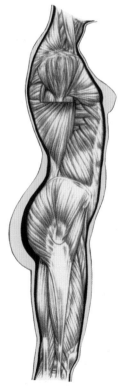

▌ The buttocks and lower back are two of the major natural fat storage areas in women.

▌ Fat distribution in women (yellow) and men (black).

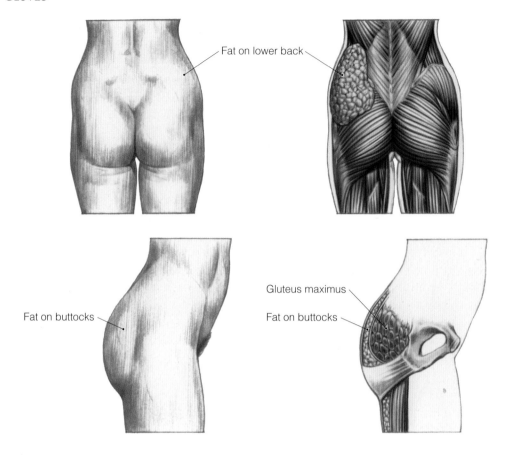

Fat on lower back

Fat on buttocks

Gluteus maximus

Fat on buttocks

Is Spot Reduction a Myth?

Is it possible to spot-reduce cellulite by specifically working the legs or the glutes? For a long time, medical studies were not able to prove that fat could be specifically eliminated in trouble spots by stimulating the underlying muscles. However, following are two major arguments in favor of the possibility of spot reduction of fat through weight or cardio training:

1. Modern studies demonstrate that exercise accelerates the use of the fat that covers the working muscles.[2]

2. Muscle contractions increase blood flow inside nearby fat stores. This accelerates the local release of fat in that specific area while preventing lipid accumulation.

In women, Heinonen measured the blood flow of the subcutaneous adipose tissue located close to the quadriceps.[3] He found that when one quadriceps was contracted by performing one leg extension, adipose blood flow increased by 200 percent over the active quadriceps, but remained completely unchanged over the inactive quadriceps.

Increasing the adipose tissue blood flow enhances the local release of fat, whereas reduced blood flow inside a fat deposit promotes its growth. Therefore, working a muscle group frequently not only prevents local fat hypertrophy but also favors the topical release of fat. Consequently, it is important to frequently contract the muscles located under the fat deposit you want to get rid of.

To accelerate fat loss on your buttocks, the stepper is the apparatus of choice provided you squeeze your buttocks together tightly throughout the exercises. To do so, you much take each step slowly to really focus on the contraction of your glutes.

At first you might have trouble maintaining this squeeze for more than a few steps. But after several workouts, you should be able to do it easily if you are concentrating. You should also lean your torso forward slightly while gently arching your lower back so that the glutes get more involved in the exercise.

However, note that the magnitude of the local fat release is small. Therefore, you will not see results in weeks, but rather, in months, unless you follow a low-calorie diet.

If you wish to develop leaner legs, you can do either cycling or running. We do not recommend swimming or rowing except for overall fat loss.

Glute Exercises

There are four main categories of exercises for the glutes from which women can benefit:

1. Hip extension
2. Bridge
3. One-leg butt press
4. Lateral hip abduction

Each category has several versions, which guarantees a great variety of movements and allows you to choose the ones that best suit both your anatomy and your goals.

Note: Squats, lunges, and deadlifts are also excellent exercises for the glutes. We do not describe them here because they are discussed in the quadriceps and hamstrings sections. To better recruit the glutes while performing these exercises, squeeze your buttocks together tightly throughout the exercises.

The goals of the warm-up sequence are to prepare the following muscles for training and reduce the risk of injury:

- Lower back
- Hips
- Quadriceps
- Hamstrings
- Calves

Perform 20 to 30 easy repetitions of the following exercises using light weights. Move from one exercise to the next without any rest. If you do not feel that one cycle was enough to warm you up, feel free to perform a second cycle.

Once you have finished this overall warm-up cycle, move on to your first glute exercise using at least one light set to specifically warm up your glutes before handling heavier weights. If you are already warmed up because you have just finished training your quadriceps or your hamstrings, there is no need to repeat the entire warm-up sequence. However, you should still do at least one set of a specific glute exercise as a warm-up.

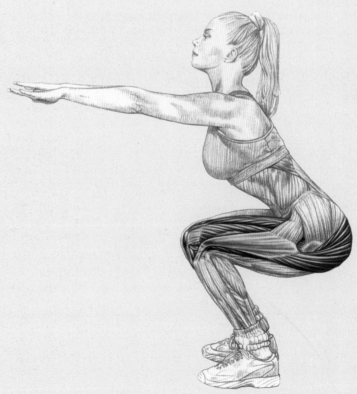

▌ **1. Squat (see page 78)**

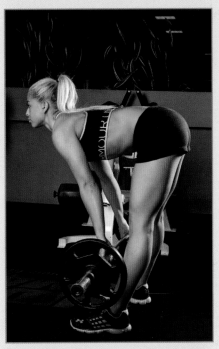

▌ 2. Stiff-leg deadlift (see page 114)

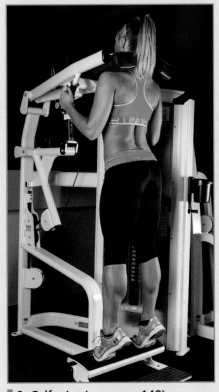

▌ 3. Calf raise (see page 143)

The hip extension belongs in the isolated, single-joint exercise category because only the hip joints are mobilized. Nevertheless, the hip extension recruits muscles in addition to the gluteus maximus: the hamstrings and the lower back.

How to Do It

Starting with both feet together, lift one leg up as far back as possible using your glutes. Hold the contracted position for one second while squeezing your buttocks together as tightly as possible. Return to the starting position and repeat. Once you have finished a set with one leg, move immediately to the other leg. To increase the range of motion, you can bring your leg forward until your thigh is about parallel with the ground and then straighten it to the back.

   The easiest way to perform the hip extension is standing because the range of motion is short and gravity results in little resistance being placed on the gluteus maximus.

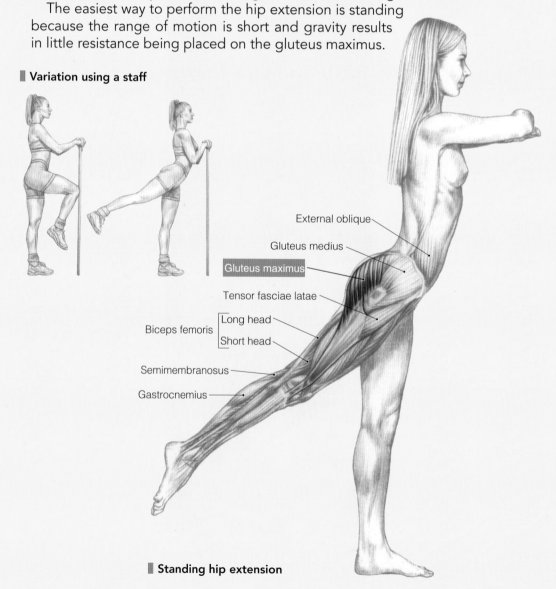

▌ **Variation using a staff**

External oblique

Gluteus medius

Gluteus maximus

Tensor fasciae latae

Biceps femoris

Long head

Short head

Semimembranosus

Gastrocnemius

▌ **Standing hip extension**

Pros

- It is the easiest exercise to perform that directly targets the glute muscles.
- It can be performed at home without much equipment.

Con

- Once you have gained more experience in weight training, you may want to move on to more complete leg exercises such as the squat or deadlift.

! **Although rounding your lower back better enables you to feel your glutes working, doing so may endanger your spine.**

Tips

- Using your free hand to touch the part of your glutes you want to develop enhances your brain–muscle connection. This simple maneuver enables you to feel your working muscles more, rendering the exercise more effective.
- You can raise your leg back only so far because the extension of the hip is limited by tension in the iliofemoral ligament (Bertin's ligament). Past a certain point, your leg will not rise anymore unless you bend your torso. Instead of moving back, it begins to move laterally. When that happens, the muscular tension is transferred from the gluteus maximus to the gluteus medius.
- To really work the gluteus maximus, do not pivot your leg toward the outside too much. It is OK for the leg to move slightly toward the outside, but do not exaggerate this abduction of the leg.

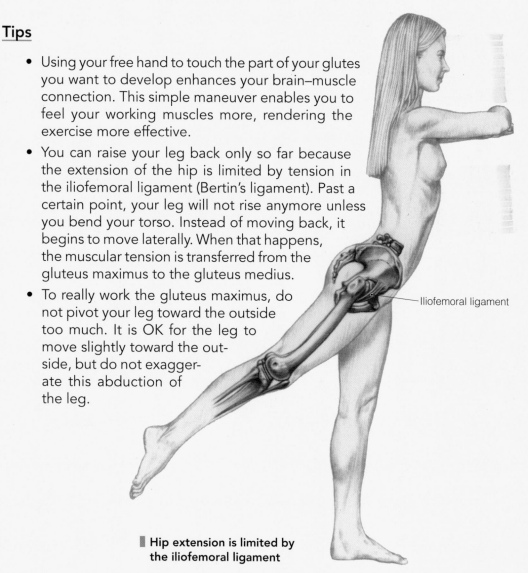

Iliofemoral ligament

▌ Hip extension is limited by the iliofemoral ligament

Standing Variations

- If you like the standing position, unless your fitness level is very low, we recommend that you not spend time performing this exercise with no resistance. You can use an elastic band, an ankle cuff weight, or an ankle cable attachment to increase the resistance.

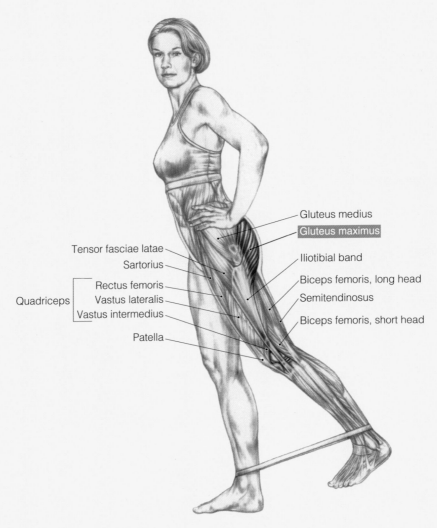

Tensor fasciae latae

Sartorius

Quadriceps — Rectus femoris
Vastus lateralis
Vastus intermedius

Patella

Gluteus medius

Gluteus maximus

Iliotibial band

Biceps femoris, long head

Semitendinosus

Biceps femoris, short head

▌ Standing variation using a resistance band

Start position

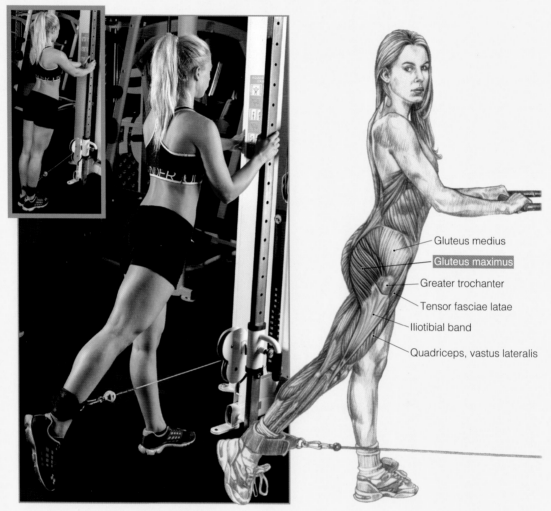

Gluteus medius

Gluteus maximus

Greater trochanter

Tensor fasciae latae

Iliotibial band

Quadriceps, vastus lateralis

Standing variation using a cable attachment

FREE WEIGHTS OR MACHINE?

All of the hip extension variations are relatively similar. Their main differences relate only to the degree of resistance placed on the glute muscles and to the range of motion of the movement. Ankle cuffs, elastic bands, and machines render the movement more effective in terms of muscle toning by adding extra resistance, thereby increasing the difficulty of the movement.

Standing Variations

- Some glute machines place extra resistance, either behind the knee or on the Achilles tendon.

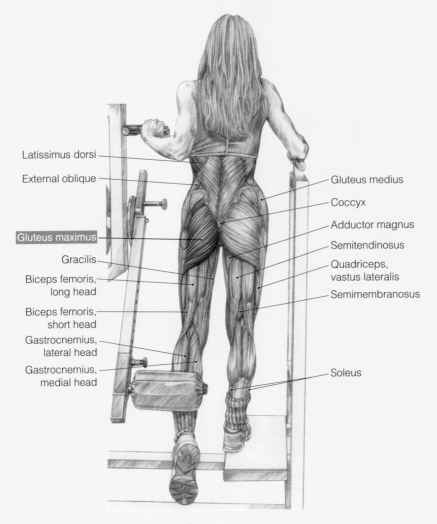

Latissimus dorsi

External oblique

Gluteus maximus

Gracilis

Biceps femoris, long head

Biceps femoris, short head

Gastrocnemius, lateral head

Gastrocnemius, medial head

Gluteus medius

Coccyx

Adductor magnus

Semitendinosus

Quadriceps, vastus lateralis

Semimembranosus

Soleus

▌ **Standing variation using a machine**

Prone Variations

By lying on the floor, you increase the resistance but decrease the range of motion.

- Lie on your abdomen and support yourself on your forearms with a slight arch in your lower back.

- You can also perform a Superman version in which you start prone with your legs out behind you and your arms straight ahead and raise your legs and arms simultaneously. This variation also works the lower back and the backs of the shoulders.

Start position

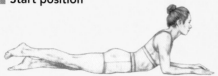

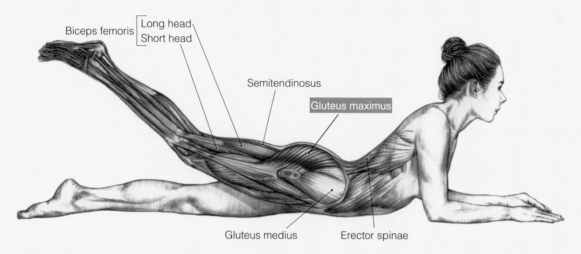

Biceps femoris — Long head
— Short head

Semitendinosus

Gluteus maximus

Gluteus medius

Erector spinae

Prone hip extension

Start position

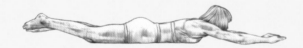

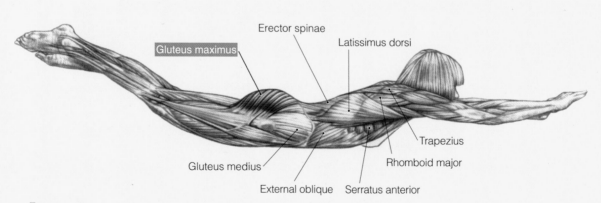

Erector spinae

Latissimus dorsi

Gluteus maximus

Gluteus medius

External oblique

Serratus anterior

Rhomboid major

Trapezius

Superman

Kneeling Variations

By kneeling, you increase both the resistance and the range of motion.

- When you bend the leg (often called a donkey kick variation), the exercise becomes easier. When you straighten it, it becomes harder. However, if you perform the exercise kneeling, you should bend your leg to 90 degrees so that you can bring it under your torso to increase the range of motion. Straighten the leg out again as soon as it is no longer underneath you. At that point, the knee joint comes into play.
- Using an elastic band, an ankle cuff weight, or an ankle cable attachment places extra weight on the glutes.

▌ The movement

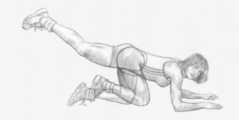

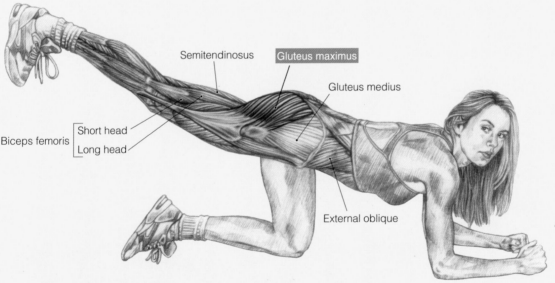

Semitendinosus

Gluteus maximus

Gluteus medius

Biceps femoris
Short head
Long head

External oblique

▌ Kneeling variation with straight leg

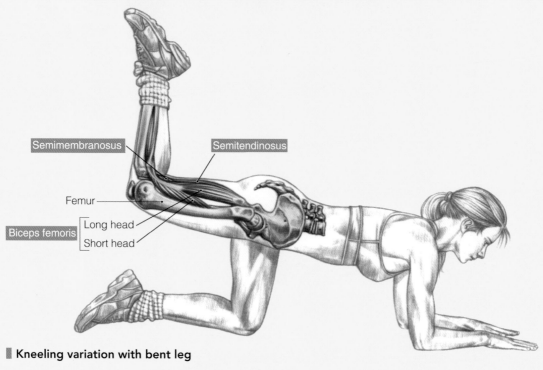

Semimembranosus

Semitendinosus

Femur

Biceps femoris — Long head / Short head

Kneeling variation with bent leg

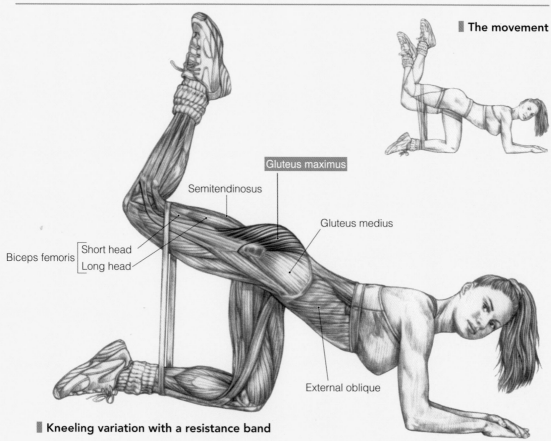

The movement

Gluteus maximus

Semitendinosus

Gluteus medius

Biceps femoris — Short head / Long head

External oblique

Kneeling variation with a resistance band

45

Kneeling Variations

- For an added challenge, positioned on your hands and knees, simultaneously lift the opposing arm and leg.
- Instead of kneeling on the floor, you can place the rested knee on a bench to further increase the range of motion of the movement and therefore its difficulty.

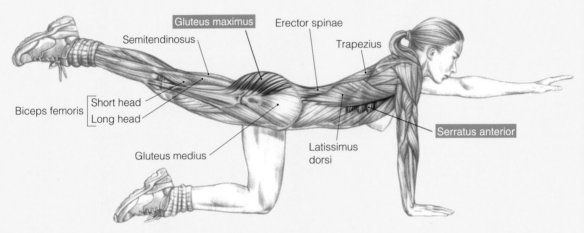

Semitendinosus

Gluteus maximus   Erector spinae

Trapezius

Biceps femoris   Short head
Long head

Gluteus medius

Latissimus dorsi

Serratus anterior

▌**Kneeling variation with opposite arm and leg raise**

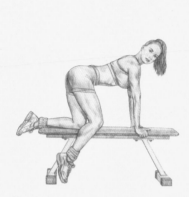

▌ **Start position**

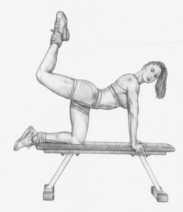

▌ **Kneeling variation on a bench; knee bent at the end of the movement**

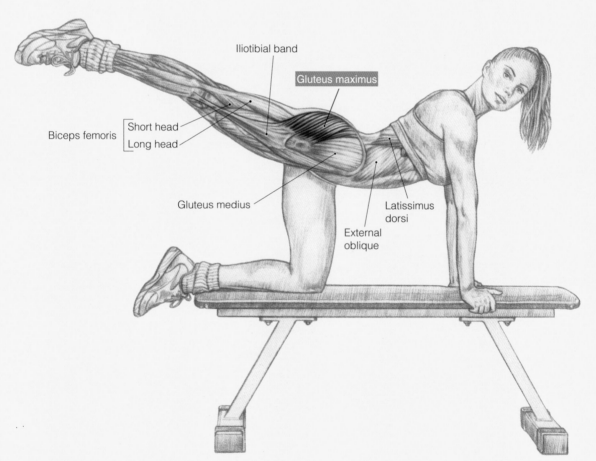

Iliotibial band

Gluteus maximus

Short head
Long head

Biceps femoris

Gluteus medius

Latissimus dorsi

External oblique

▌ **Kneeling variation on a bench; knee straight at the end of the movement**

Machine Variation

- Machines called Butt Blasters add extra resistance on the soles of your feet to render the exercise more intense and more effective. Note that there is a difference in the movement because the knee joint is mobilized. As a result, in addition to recruiting the glutes and the hamstrings, the quadriceps also come into play.

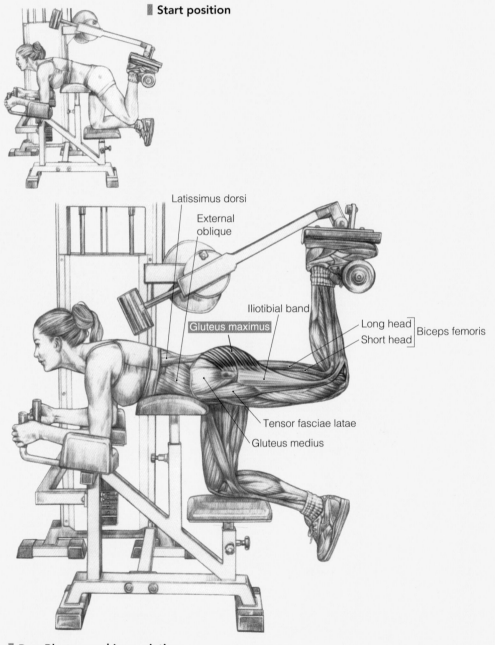

▌ **Start position**

Latissimus dorsi

External oblique

Iliotibial band

Gluteus maximus

Long head ⎤
Short head ⎦ Biceps femoris

Tensor fasciae latae

Gluteus medius

▌ **Butt Blaster machine variation**

The bridge belongs in the basic, multiple-joint exercise category because the hip, knee, and ankle joints are mobilized. As a result, the bridge recruits muscles in addition to the glutes: the lumbar muscles and thighs.

How to Do It

Lie on your back with your knees bent at 90 degrees. Place your arms by your sides. Using your shoulders as a pivot point, raise your torso by contracting your glutes as tightly as possible while pushing on your heels. Hold the contracted position for one second before returning to the starting position. Make sure you use constant tension by stopping each repetition short of touching the floor with your glutes.

▌ **Start position**

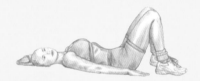

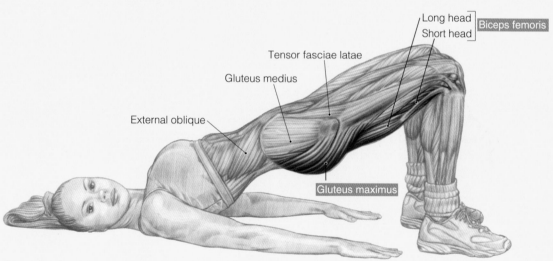

Long head ⎤
Short head ⎦ Biceps femoris

Tensor fasciae latae

Gluteus medius

External oblique

Gluteus maximus

▌ **Two-leg bridge**

Pros

- It is a very easy exercise to perform to tone your whole legs, especially the glute muscles.
- It can be performed at home without much equipment.

Con

- You will progress very quickly, which will force you to find ways to render this exercise more challenging.

(!) Keep your lower back really straight. If you overextend it, you may damage your discs.

Tips

- Place your hands on the sides of your glutes to better feel them working.
- To increase your range of motion, don't arch your lower back too much.
- Unlike the woman modeling this exercise in the illustrations, you should not turn your head to the side. Rather, look at the ceiling so that you do not damage your cervical spine.

FREE WEIGHTS OR MACHINE?

No machine can duplicate this body weight exercise. Fortunately, there are several ways to increase the resistance placed on your muscles to make this movement even more effective.

Variations

When this exercise becomes too easy, you may render it more effective by doing any of the following:

- Add an extra load on your body by placing a weight on the lower part of your abdomen.
- Lift one leg.
- Place your calves or feet on a bench or chair to achieve a greater range of motion requiring a more powerful muscle contraction.

▎Start position

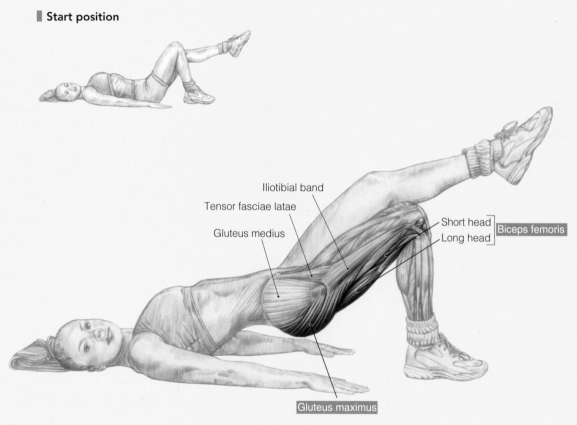

Iliotibial band

Tensor fasciae latae

Gluteus medius

Short head — Biceps femoris
Long head

Gluteus maximus

▎One-leg bridge

Variations

▮ Bridge with calves on a bench

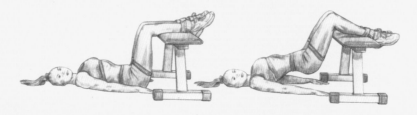

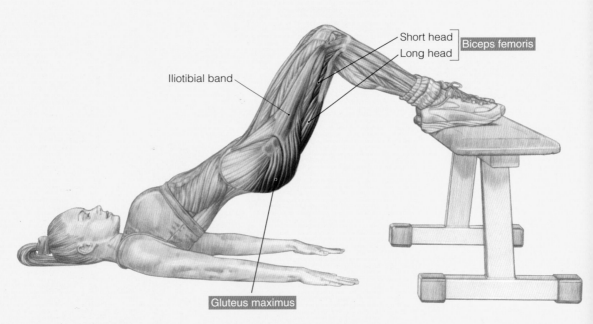

Short head
Long head
Biceps femoris

Iliotibial band

Gluteus maximus

▮ Bridge with feet on a bench

The butt press belongs in the basic, multiple-joint exercise category because the hip, knee, and ankle joints are all mobilized. As a result, the butt press recruits muscles in addition to the glutes: the lumbar muscles and thighs. This movement requires the use of the assisted pull-up machine to target the glutes very effectively.

How to Do It

Firmly grab the dip bars or machine supports to ensure stability. Instead of kneeling on the pad of the assisted pull-up machine, place one foot on it. Keep the other foot firmly on the foot step or the floor. Press on the assistant lever, squeezing your glutes as tightly as possible. Do not straighten your leg completely so that your glutes remain in a constant state of tension before you return to the starting position and repeat. When you have finished a set with one leg, move immediately to the other leg.

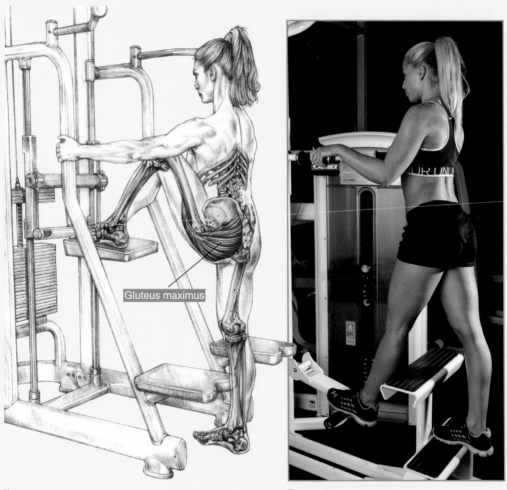

Gluteus maximus

▌ **Start position**   ▌ **One-leg butt press**

Pro

- This exercise stretches your glutes like no others can. You will feel them contract immediately.

Con

- You have to work one leg at a time, which makes this exercise more time-consuming than bilateral exercises.

 Because it is unilateral, this exercise places an uneven pressure on your lower back, which might exacerbate any existing pain or damage.

Tips

- If your hamstrings or ankles are not flexible enough, they will limit your range of motion, rendering this exercise less effective. Therefore, it is a good idea to stretch them both before starting this movement.
- Do not arch your back too much as you straighten your leg in an attempt to get a more powerful contraction of the glutes. If your back is pain free, a little arching of the lower back is fine, but excessive arching can damage your discs.
- By controlling how high the machine raises your working leg, you can modulate the range of motion of the exercise. At first, to prevent unnecessary soreness, do not let your foot go too high in the stretching part of the movement. Once you are used to this exercise, your goal should be to get the longest range of motion possible by letting the machine bring your foot as high as possible to really stretch your glutes.

Variation

If you don't have access to an assisted pull-up machine, you can perform a one-leg step up, which is also described as a lunge variation in the quadriceps section. However, the butt press is preferable for two main reasons:

1. You benefit from a greater range of motion because of the deeper stretch provided by the butt press.
2. It is far easier to adjust the degree of resistance with the butt press, which is important when you first start training. With the step-up, you are forced to lift at least almost your entire body weight at a minimum.

▊ Start position

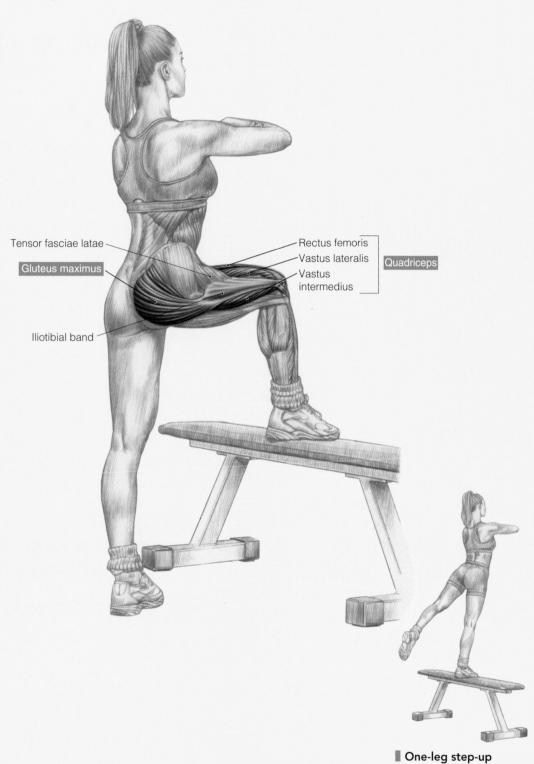

Tensor fasciae latae

Gluteus maximus

Iliotibial band

Rectus femoris

Vastus lateralis

Vastus intermedius

Quadriceps

▊ One-leg step-up

55

LATERAL HIP ABDUCTION

The lateral hip abduction belongs in the isolated, single-joint exercise category because only the hip joints are mobilized. As a consequence, the lateral hip abduction does not recruit muscles other than its primary targets: the gluteus medius and the gluteus minimus.

How to Do It

Lie on your side with your bottom hand either flat on the floor or supporting your head and your top hand resting on the floor. By contracting your glutes, raise your leg as high as possible. Hold this contraction for a count of 2 before lowering your leg. Make sure you use constant tension by stopping each repetition short of your legs touching each other. Keep your body, especially your legs, straight at all times throughout the exercise.

By lying laterally on the floor, you increase the resistance but decrease the range of motion. The working leg can be either kept straight (harder version) or bent (easier version).

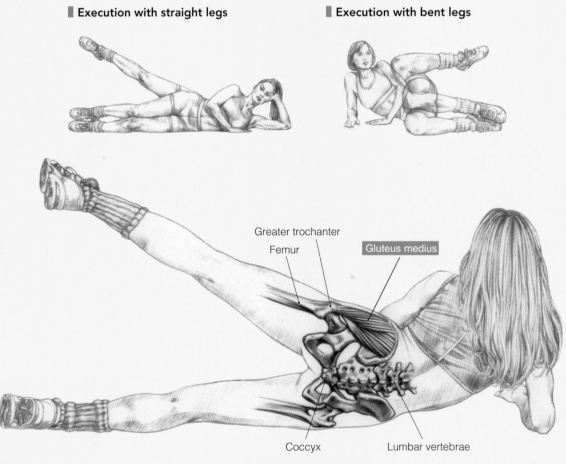

▎**Execution with straight legs**

▎**Execution with bent legs**

Greater trochanter

Femur

Gluteus medius

Coccyx

Lumbar vertebrae

▎**Lateral hip abduction**

Changing your leg position changes the area of the buttocks that is targeted.

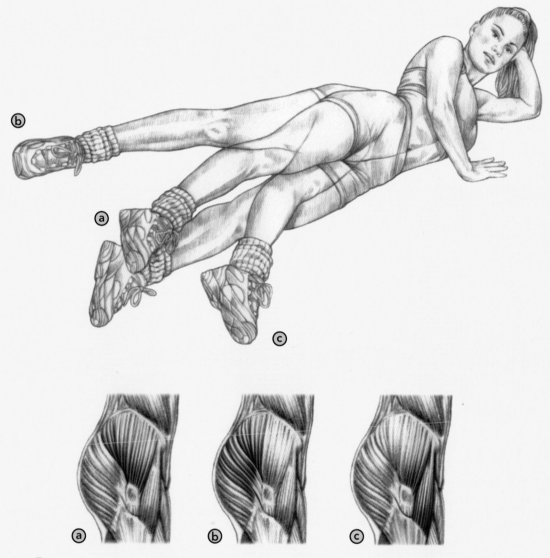

Three leg positions and the corresponding targeted buttocks areas: *(a)* vertical, *(b)* slightly back, *(c)* slightly forward

LATERAL HIP ABDUCTION

By using an elastic band, an ankle cuff weight, or an ankle cable attachment, you can apply extra resistance to the gluteus medius.

▌ Start position

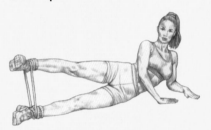

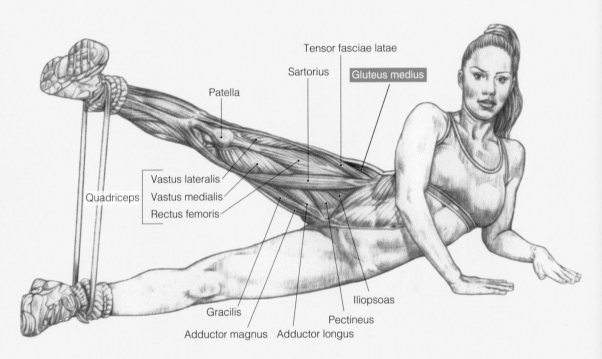

Tensor fasciae latae

Sartorius

Gluteus medius

Patella

Vastus lateralis

Quadriceps — Vastus medialis

Rectus femoris

Gracilis

Adductor magnus   Adductor longus

Pectineus

Iliopsoas

▌ Variation using a resistance band

Pro

- Studies have shown that the lateral hip abduction is the best exercise to target the gluteus medius, the toning of which provides a rounder appearance to your glutes.[4]

Con

- This exercise works only a tiny portion of the glutes. As a result, it should make up only a small fraction of your glute workout.

- **When performed in a unilateral fashion, this exercise might place an uneven pressure on your lower back, which could exacerbate any existing pain.**
- **Arching your back allows a greater range of motion, but this is dangerous for your lower back.**

Tips

- If your knees shake laterally during squats or lunges, your abductor muscles are too weak. Abductor exercises will correct this problem and therefore better protect your knees.
- Using your free hand to touch the part of your glutes you want to develop enhances your brain–muscle connection. This simple maneuver enables you to feel your working muscles more, rendering the exercise more effective.
- You can elevate your leg laterally only so far. Some women have a greater range of motion than others. This is *not* due to greater flexibility, but rather to the shape of their bones. It is not a good idea to try to go past your natural range of motion because doing so could damage your hip joint.

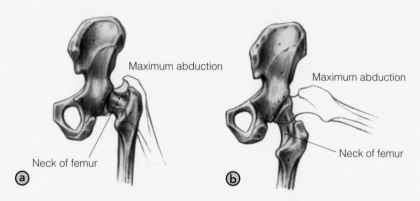

(a) This femur does not have much room to rise because of the limited space offered by a curved pelvis cup. *(b)* This femur has plenty of room to rise because of the large space offered by a flat pelvis cup.

Standing Variations

The easiest way to perform the lateral hip abduction is standing because the range of motion is short and gravity results in little resistance placed on the gluteus medius.

▌ **Standing variation using a staff**

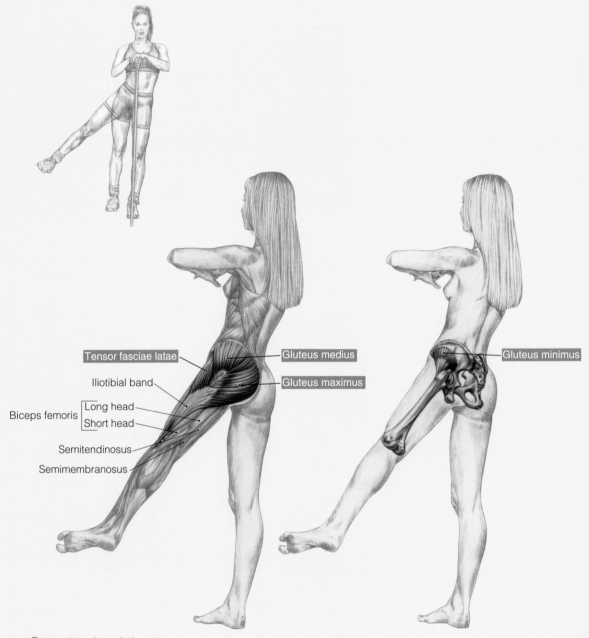

Tensor fasciae latae

Gluteus medius

Iliotibial band

Gluteus maximus

Biceps femoris

Long head

Short head

Gluteus minimus

Semitendinosus

Semimembranosus

▌ **Standing hip abduction**

If you like the standing position, unless your fitness level is very low, we recommend that you not spend time on this version with no resistance. You can use an elastic band, an ankle cuff weight, or an ankle cable attachment to increase the resistance.

▊ The movement

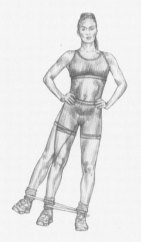

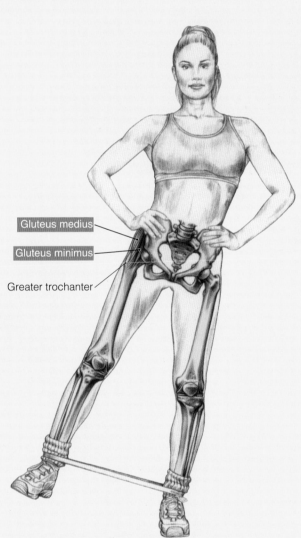

Gluteus medius

Gluteus minimus

Greater trochanter

▊ **Standing variation using a resistance band**

LATERAL HIP ABDUCTION

Standing Variations

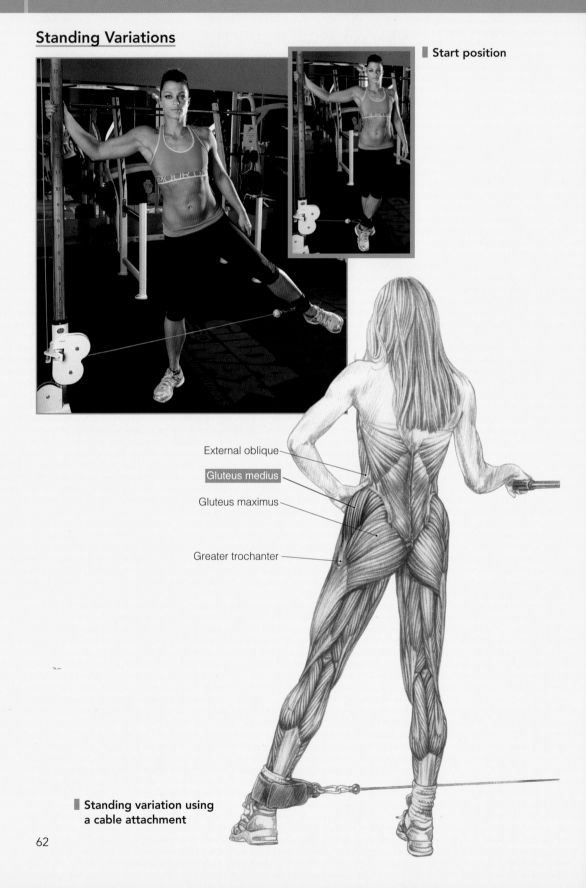

External oblique

Gluteus medius

Gluteus maximus

Greater trochanter

Standing variation using
a cable attachment

62

Kneeling Variation

By kneeling, you increase both the resistance and the range of motion. In the kneeling version, you have to bend your leg to move it up laterally.

▌ **Start position**

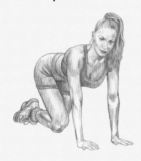

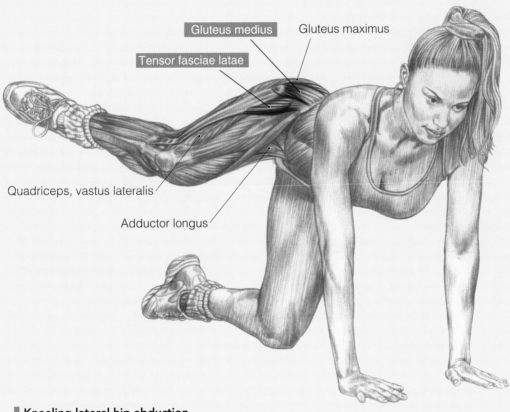

Gluteus medius

Gluteus maximus

Tensor fasciae latae

Quadriceps, vastus lateralis

Adductor longus

▌ **Kneeling lateral hip abduction**

Machine Variations

Two kinds of machines are available to increase the resistance on your legs and make the exercise more effective.

- One, in which you are seated, allows you to work both legs simultaneously. By bending forward or backward on the seated machine, you can shift the area of the glutes that experiences the majority of the contraction. By bending backward, you favor the recruitment of the upper area of the external part of the glutes. By bending forward, you favor the recruitment of the middle area of the external part of the glutes.

▌Start position

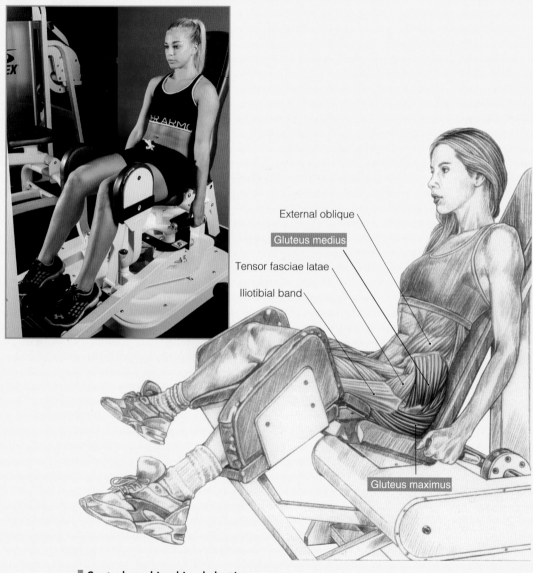

External oblique

Gluteus medius

Tensor fasciae latae

Iliotibial band

Gluteus maximus

▌**Seated machine hip abduction**

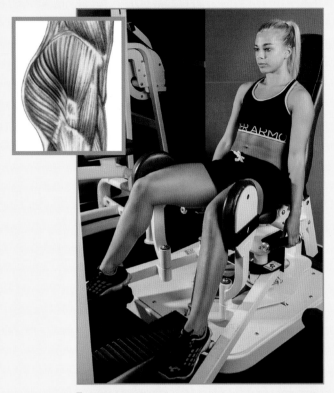

Backward lean

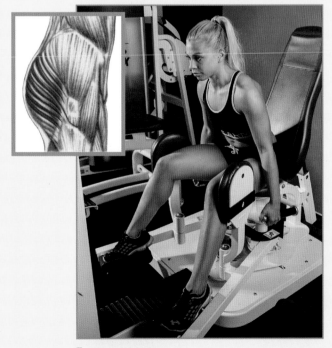

Forward lean

Machine Variations

- The other machine allows you to train in a standing position. Some standing machines allow you to train both legs at a time; whereas others, only one. In both versions, the movement is the same as that of the other variations.

FREE WEIGHTS OR MACHINE?

All of the lateral hip abduction variations are relatively similar. Their main differences relate only to the degree of resistance placed on the glute muscles and to the range of motion of the movement. Ankle cuffs, elastic bands, and machines render the movement more effective in terms of muscle toning by adding extra resistance, thereby increasing the difficulty of the movement.

Some abductor machines have you keep your legs straight, whereas others have you bend your legs to 90 degrees. If you are a beginner, these latter machines are preferable for the following reasons:

- You are less likely to overstretch your abductor muscles with your legs bent.
- They are gentler on the knees.
- Your leg muscles are placed in a stronger position so you can handle heavier weight.

▌ The movement

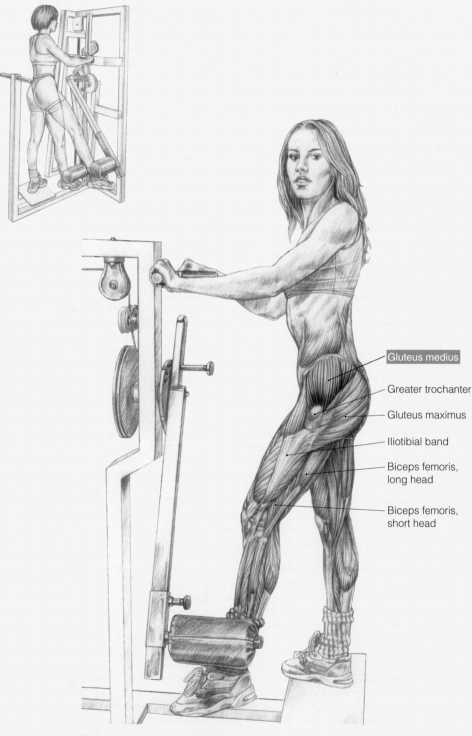

Gluteus medius

Greater trochanter

Gluteus maximus

Iliotibial band

Biceps femoris, long head

Biceps femoris, short head

▌ Standing machine hip abduction

- Lunges (see the quadriceps section for details) are an excellent way to stretch the glutes. Instead of putting your foot on the floor in front of you, you could put it on a bench to increase the range of the stretch. For best use of this range of motion, bend your back leg so that you can drop your buttocks lower than your elevated foot. Hold the stretching position for 10 to 20 seconds. Lunge backward and repeat immediately with the other leg.

- Note that, in general, exercises that stretch the hamstrings also increase flexibility in the glutes. For another stretch, lie on your back on the floor and grab one leg with your hands to bring it closer to your torso while bending it (easier version) or keeping it straight (advanced version). Hold the stretching position for 20 to 30 seconds. Once one glute has been stretched, repeat immediately with the other leg.

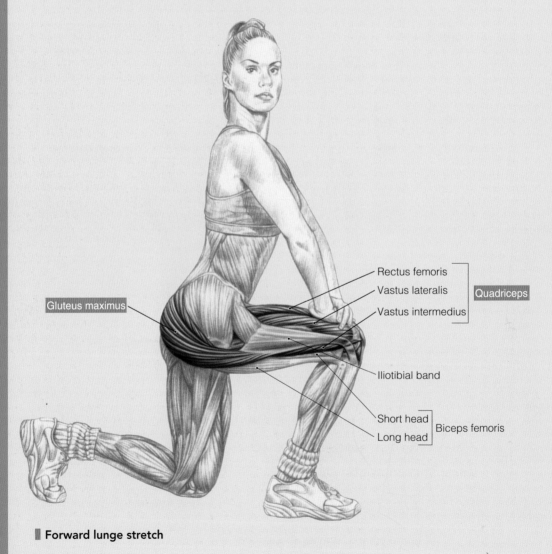

▌ **Forward lunge stretch**

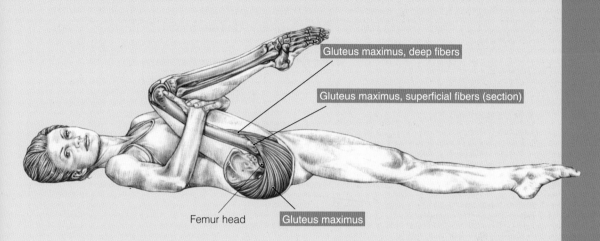

Gluteus maximus, deep fibers

Gluteus maximus, superficial fibers (section)

Femur head

Gluteus maximus

▌ Glute and hamstring stretch with leg bent

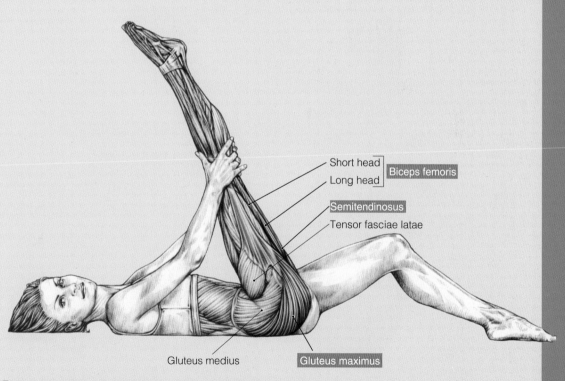

Short head | Biceps femoris
Long head

Semitendinosus

Tensor fasciae latae

Gluteus medius

Gluteus maximus

▌ Glute and hamstring stretch with leg straight

- For a seated stretch, sit on the floor with one leg straight. Bend the other leg and place it over the other. Push your knee toward your chest with your elbow, bringing the bent leg as close as possible to your torso. Hold the stretching position for 10 to 20 seconds. Once one glute has been stretched, repeat immediately with the other leg.

▌Start position

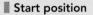

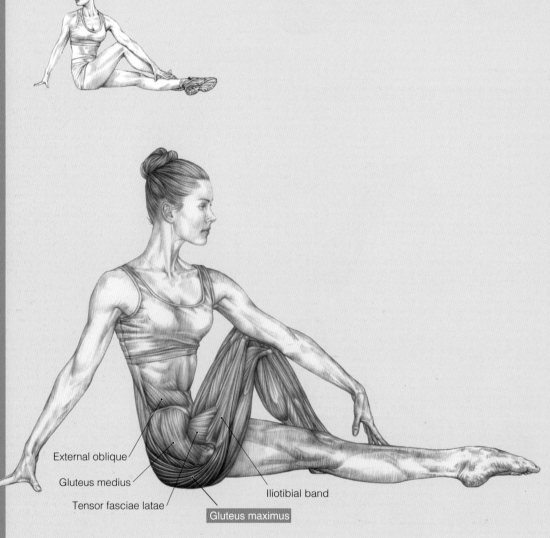

External oblique

Gluteus medius

Tensor fasciae latae

Iliotibial band

Gluteus maximus

▌Seated glute stretch

The rotator muscles of the hips play an important role in maintaining the proper curve in the lumbar spine. When these muscles are not flexible enough, they pull the lower back forward, making the lumbar spine lose its natural curve. This misalignment renders the intervertebral discs very vulnerable to the jolts normally experienced when standing or walking. Stretching the rotator muscles of the hips is particularly important to prevent back problems and injuries, especially in athletes.[5]

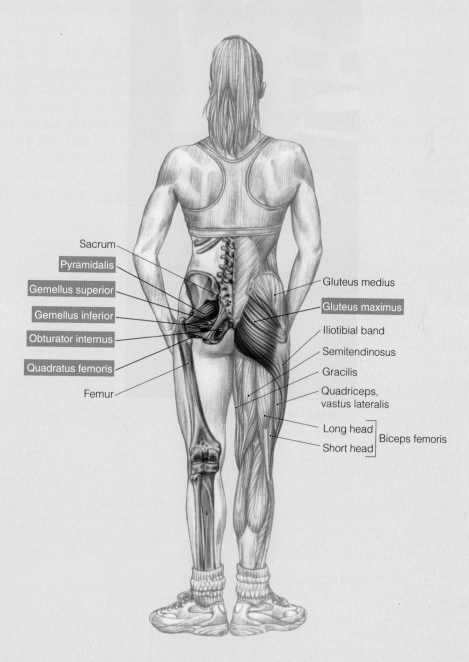

Sacrum

Pyramidalis

Gemellus superior

Gemellus inferior

Obturator internus

Quadratus femoris

Femur

Gluteus medius

Gluteus maximus

Iliotibial band

Semitendinosus

Gracilis

Quadriceps, vastus lateralis

Long head ⎤
Short head ⎦ Biceps femoris

SQUAT

The squat belongs in the basic, multiple-joint exercise category because the hip, knee, and ankle joints are mobilized. As a result, the squat recruits many muscles in addition to the quadriceps: the glutes, hamstrings, lumbar muscles, and calves.

The squat is considered a good starting exercise because it stimulates many muscle groups of the lower body.

How to Do It

Stand with your feet about shoulder-width apart, and place a barbell on your upper back. Keeping your back arched very slightly backward, bend your legs just until your torso starts to really bend forward. When this happens, thigh involvement lessens and the lumbar muscles begin to do the majority of the work.

When you have reached your low position, push down through your heels to straighten your legs. Once you are upright, perform another repetition.

Pro

- The whole lower-body and part of the upper-body muscles are recruited, which makes the squat one of the most complete exercises.

Con

- The squat is a very difficult exercise to perform and requires athletic skills a beginner may not have.

Because this exercise is exhausting, it carries some risk for the knees and back. Hanging at a pull-up bar to stretch your spine after your workout is advised, as it is with every workout.

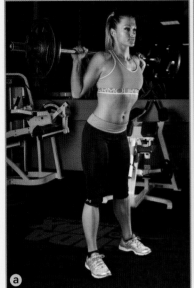
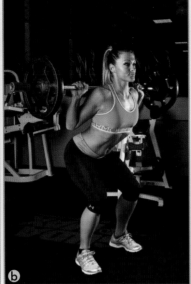
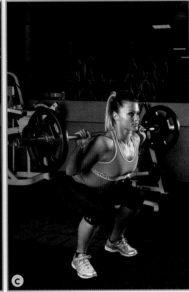

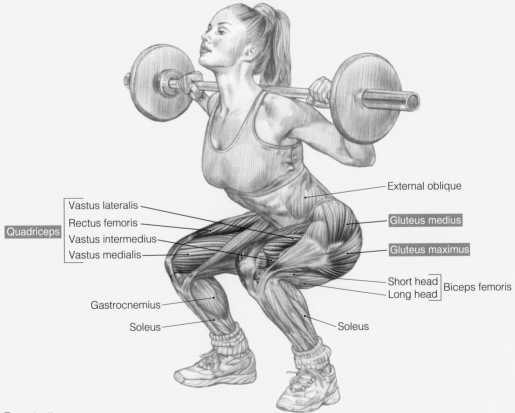

Quadriceps

Vastus lateralis

Rectus femoris

Vastus intermedius

Vastus medialis

Gastrocnemius

Soleus

External oblique

Gluteus medius

Gluteus maximus

Short head
Long head — Biceps femoris

Soleus

▎ Barbell squat

Tips

- Whenever you use a barbell, do not place it on your neck because doing so is likely to hurt your spine. Place the bar below your neck, roughly at your rear shoulder level. If the bar hurts, put a towel around it to make it more comfortable.

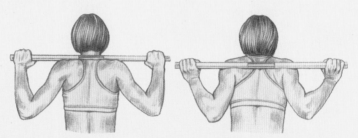

▌Hold the bar on your trapezius and the top of your shoulders (left) or across the back of your shoulders and trapezius (right).

- In order to increase the muscular intensity of the squat, use a continuous tension technique. This means that instead of allowing your leg muscles to rest at the top of the movement by completely straightening your legs, you stop your squat short and don't straighten your legs completely. Perform as many repetitions as possible using continuous tension. When the burn becomes unbearable, straighten your legs at the top of the movement in order to give your muscles a short rest, which will allow you to perform a few extra reps.

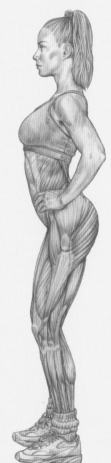

▌Keep your legs slightly bent at the top of the squat to make the exercise more difficult.

- Placing a thin board of wood or a weight plate under your heels will make it easier to keep your back straight as you go down. This trick is particularly helpful if you have long femurs or inflexible ankles.

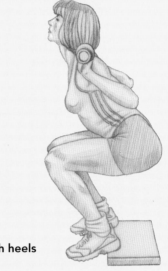

▌ Squat with heels elevated

- If you have a recurvatum (hyperextension) at the knee level (you can straighten your legs so far that your knees are pushed backward), *do not* straighten your legs at all because the load can damage your knees in that precarious position. Worse, your legs could bend backward under the load, which would result in very serious injuries.

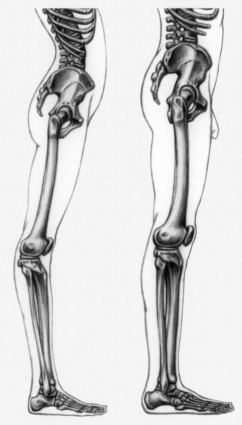

▌ Hyperextension (left) is typical of women; straighter legs (right) are typical of men.

- In order to protect your spine from excessive damaging pressure, as your muscles grow stronger, we recommend that you don't perform both squats and deadlifts during the same workout. As you advance in your training, center your leg workouts around squats and save the deadlifts for your back workouts.

- Do not look down or to the side when performing a squat. Rather, look in front of you and slightly up to avoid damaging your neck.

- Rounding your back, especially at the end of a set when your muscles are tired, is much easier than keeping your back straight, but this rounded position increases the risk of damaging your lumbar discs.

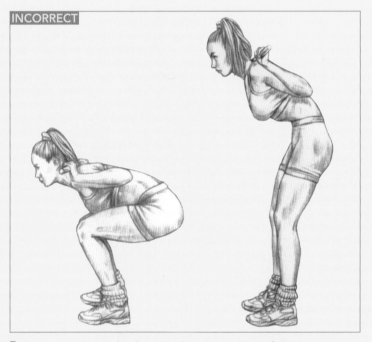

INCORRECT

▌ **Don't round your back at the bottom or top of the movement.**

Stance Width

Varying the width of your feet during the squat can change the muscles targeted. Keeping them at about shoulder width and slightly turned out results in the muscles of the entire thigh doing equal work. When you narrow your stance, the focus is on the quadriceps, and the knee joints experience greater pressure. Adopting a very wide stance works the inner thighs, hamstrings, and glutes more. As with all variations, choose the one that feels most natural to you at first. Later, you can adopt a position that targets particular muscular zones.

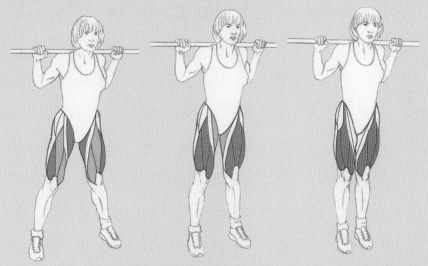

Comparison of wide, shoulder-width, and narrow stances for the squat. Red illustrates the muscles that are most engaged, orange illustrates those that are less engaged.

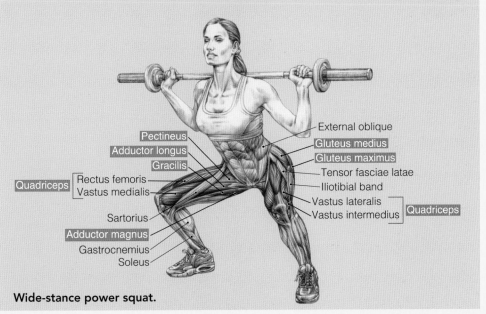

Pectineus
Adductor longus
Gracilis
Quadriceps
Rectus femoris
Vastus medialis
Sartorius
Adductor magnus
Gastrocnemius
Soleus

External oblique
Gluteus medius
Gluteus maximus
Tensor fasciae latae
Iliotibial band
Vastus lateralis
Vastus intermedius
Quadriceps

Wide-stance power squat.

Body Weight Variations

- The easiest squat version is the free squat, in which you use only your own body weight. You can practice this exercise at home to tone up your legs without having to go to the gym. The main problem is that body weight squats rapidly become too easy because of the lack of resistance.

▌ Start position

▌ Variations with arms crossed in front or down at the sides. Choose the arm position that feels the most comfortable and secure for you; arm position does not alter the recruitment of the leg muscles.

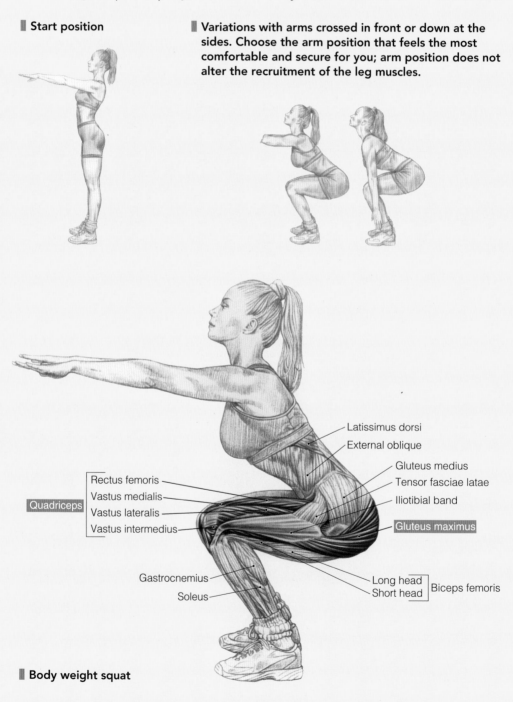

Latissimus dorsi

External oblique

Gluteus medius

Tensor fasciae latae

Iliotibial band

Rectus femoris

Vastus medialis

Quadriceps

Vastus lateralis

Vastus intermedius

Gluteus maximus

Gastrocnemius

Soleus

Long head

Short head

Biceps femoris

▌ Body weight squat

- Alternatively, you can do one-leg squats, which are much harder than regular squats and do not put pressure on the spine. If this variation is new to you, make sure you control the degree of descent, because the maximal range of motion of the one-leg squat can be much greater than that of the regular squat. Going as deep as possible may result in profound muscular soreness after your workout. Therefore, increase your range of motion gradually over several workouts.

▌ Start position

▌ Variation with one leg in front and arms straight out; this will train your balance as well as your muscles.

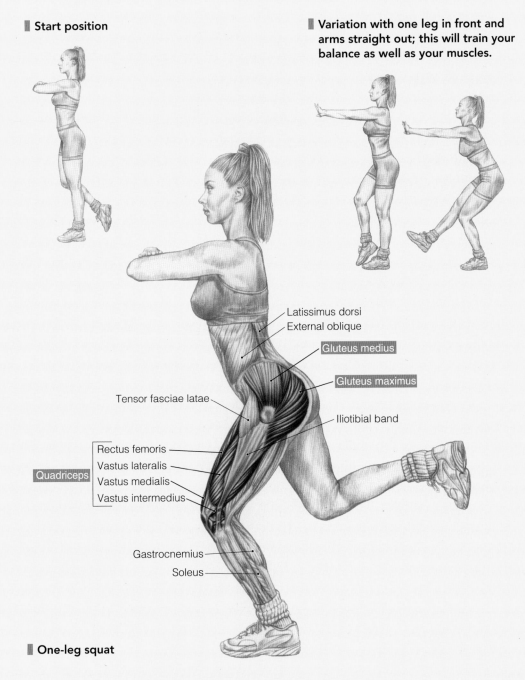

Latissimus dorsi
External oblique
Gluteus medius
Gluteus maximus
Tensor fasciae latae
Iliotibial band
Rectus femoris
Vastus lateralis
Quadriceps
Vastus medialis
Vastus intermedius
Gastrocnemius
Soleus

▌ One-leg squat

85

Squat Depth

The deeper you lower the weight, the more intense the squat becomes, because as you increase your range of motion, you are not recruiting only your quadriceps. Your hamstrings and especially your buttocks are going to be heavily recruited, as well. So, it seems to be a good idea to squat deep. From a muscular stand point, this is correct. But this is also where your morphology will come into play. The taller you are, the more you will have to bend your torso forward in order to keep your equilibrium as you squat down. In this position, the risk of spinal injury increases dramatically.

Many people claim that bending the torso forward during a squat is bad technique. But morphologically, if you have long quadriceps and a shorter torso, it is mechanically impossible to keep your back straight as you go down in squats. You must bend forward to keep your balance. This is why it is easier to keep your back straight using a Smith machine because there is no balance issue!

If you find that you have to bend forward to a dangerous level in free squats, you would be wise to find an alternative to this exercise rather than waste hours trying to master a technique that you cannot perform morphologically.

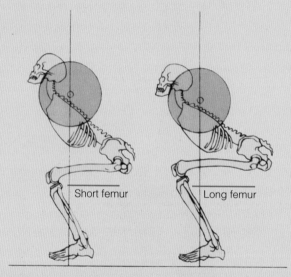

Short femur   Long femur

Short femurs mean less forward lean; long femurs mean more forward lean. The longer your femur is, the more you will have to bend over to keep your equilibrium. Therefore, as a general rule, the taller you are, the more dangerous it is for your spine to squat deep.

Dumbbell Variations

- When you grab one dumbbell between your legs, your thighs have to work harder, rendering the squat more effective. As an alternative, you can use a strong elastic band or squat on one leg only.

▌ Start position

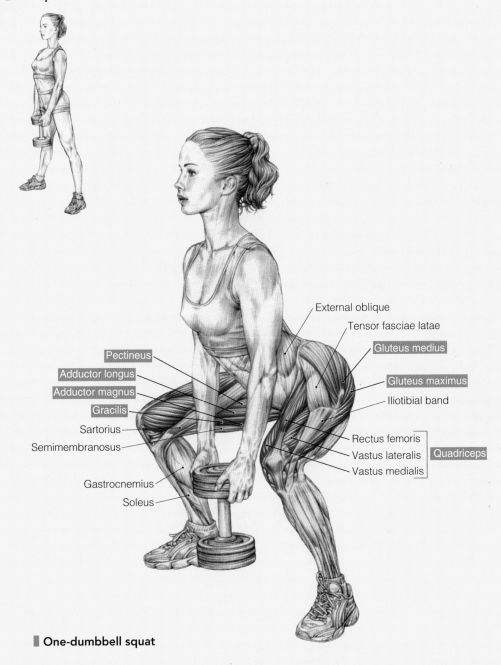

External oblique

Tensor fasciae latae

Gluteus medius

Pectineus

Adductor longus

Adductor magnus

Gracilis

Sartorius

Semimembranosus

Gluteus maximus

Iliotibial band

Rectus femoris

Vastus lateralis

Vastus medialis

Quadriceps

Gastrocnemius

Soleus

▌ One-dumbbell squat

Dumbbell Variations

- Grabbing two dumbbells adds even more resistance. The main advantage of dumbbells over a barbell is that they make it easier to keep your back straight and to keep your balance. However, as you grow stronger, dumbbells will not offer the resistance required to progress even more. This is when graduating to a long bar is required. By then, you should be able to keep your balance despite the overload placed on your legs.

▌ **Start position**

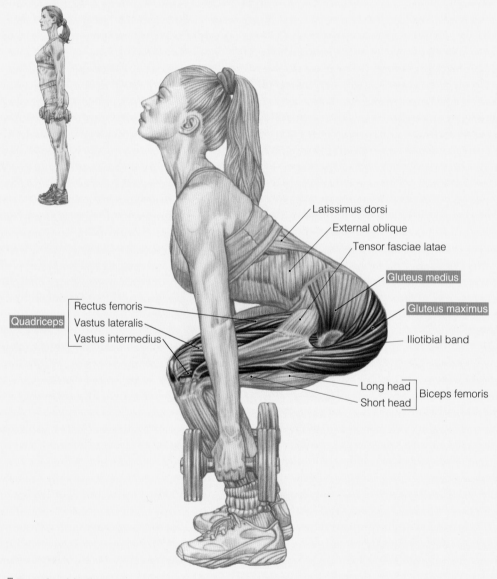

Latissimus dorsi
External oblique
Tensor fasciae latae
Gluteus medius
Gluteus maximus
Iliotibial band
Rectus femoris
Quadriceps
Vastus lateralis
Vastus intermedius
Long head
Short head
Biceps femoris

▌ **Two-dumbbell squat**

Resistance Band Variation

- An elastic band can replace dumbbells. The main advantage of the resistance band is that it provides a variable resistance that suits your muscular strength exactly. At the bottom of the movement, where your muscles are weaker, the band offers less resistance. As you straighten your legs and your muscles get stronger, the band gets pulled and therefore offers more resistance.

▌ Start position

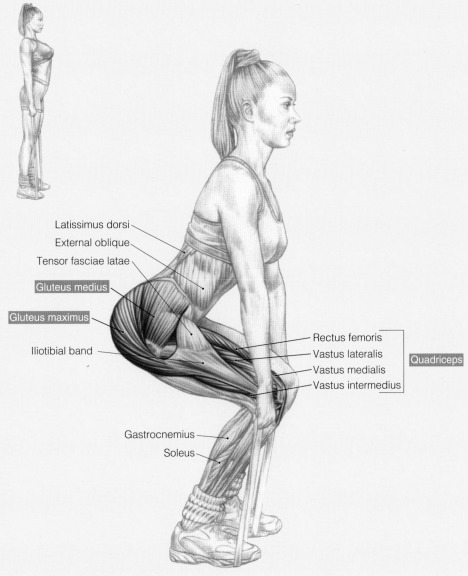

Latissimus dorsi
External oblique
Tensor fasciae latae
Gluteus medius
Gluteus maximus
Iliotibial band

Rectus femoris
Vastus lateralis
Vastus medialis
Vastus intermedius
Quadriceps

Gastrocnemius
Soleus

▌ Squat using a resistance band

Front Squat Variation

- The front squat allows you to keep your back straighter than you can with the classic back squat. However, it shifts the muscular recruitment from the glutes to the quadriceps, which may not be your goal if your main focus is glute development. Furthermore, carrying the bar on the front shoulders will feel very uncomfortable for many women. Moreover, mastering proper front squat technique is difficult. Without it, you will be very prone to losing your balance. As a result of these problems, the front squat is not a top leg exercise for most women.

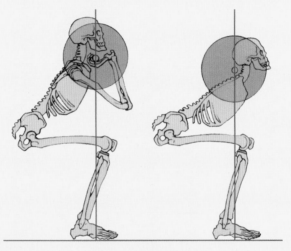

▍Compared to the back squat (on the right), the front squat allows you to keep a straighter back.

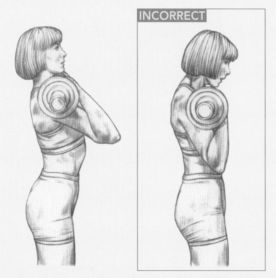

▍On the left, proper bar placement technique with the elbows elevated. On the right, improper bar placement technique with the elbows down.

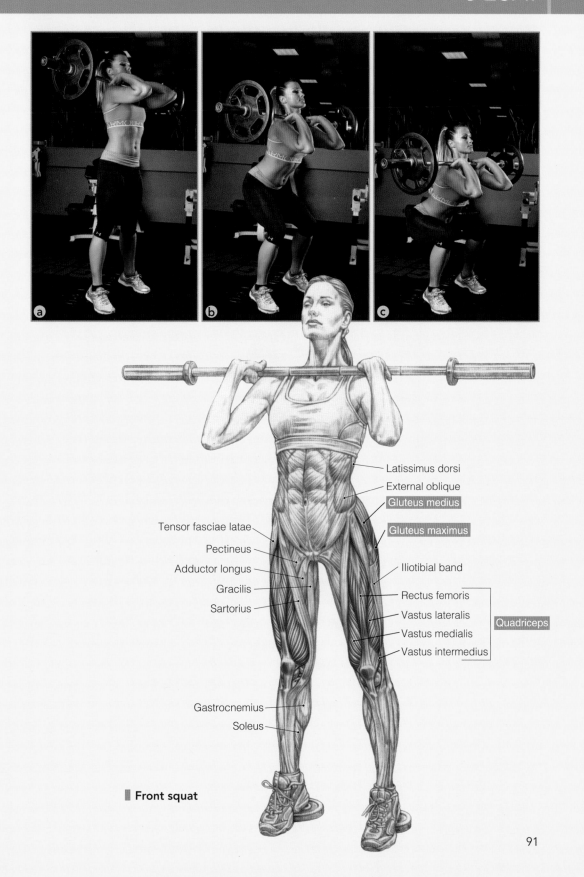

Latissimus dorsi

External oblique

Gluteus medius

Gluteus maximus

Tensor fasciae latae

Iliotibial band

Pectineus

Adductor longus

Rectus femoris

Gracilis

Vastus lateralis

Sartorius

Vastus medialis

Quadriceps

Vastus intermedius

Gastrocnemius

Soleus

▌ Front squat

Smith Machine Variation

- Smith machines can be a good substitute for free-weight squats because the guidance they offer reduces the likelihood of accident due to a loss of balance. On a Smith machine you can place your feet forward, which allows you to keep your back very straight. In that position, you are recruiting your glutes while sparing your spine and your knees. An attempt to adopt such a position in a free squat will cause you to fall backward. Because of the stability of the Smith machine, you can easily keep your balance. Therefore, it is an excellent substitute for free squats, especially for beginners.

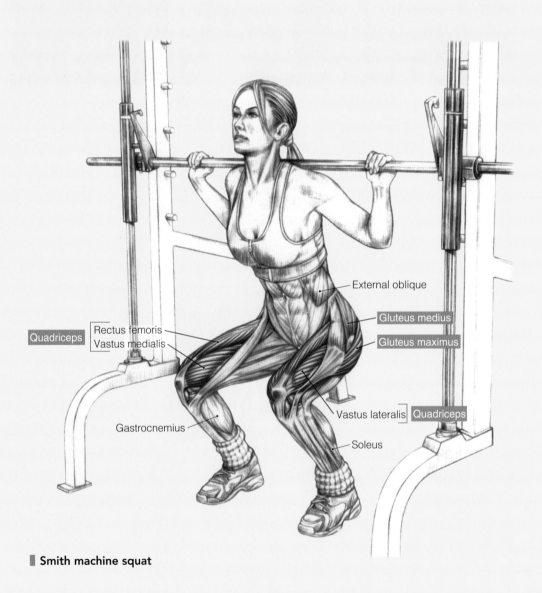

▌ **Smith machine squat**

The Smith machine also allows you to adopt just about every foot position you wish to better target the areas of your lower body you want. Following are foot positions and the muscles they tend to recruit:

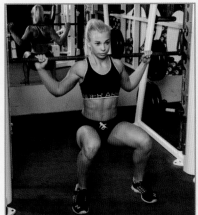

Forward: glutes and hamstrings

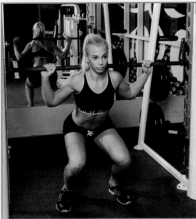

Under the glutes: quadriceps (this position is tougher on your knees)

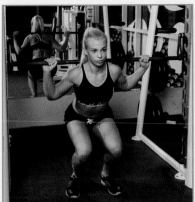

Together: quadriceps

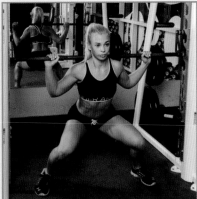

Wide apart: adductors

FREE WEIGHTS OR MACHINE?

There are plenty of squat machines. Their main advantage is that they are less hazardous than the free squat because you have no degree of freedom in terms of the trajectory of the movement. Therefore, it is much harder to lose your balance. This is especially important for beginners with no athletic background. However, this very rigid trajectory is also the Achilles' heel of squat machines, because they do not suit most women's morphology. If a machine does not fit yours, your back is likely to end up in a very awkward position. Therefore, it is hard to recommend squat machines. If you wish to train on a leg machine that spares your back, it is better to use a leg press than a squat machine.

Other Machine Variations

- The hack squat places less pressure on the spine, but it is designed to optimize the recruitment of the quadriceps while minimizing that of the glutes. As a result, it may not suit you if you are more interested in working the glutes.

▌ The movement

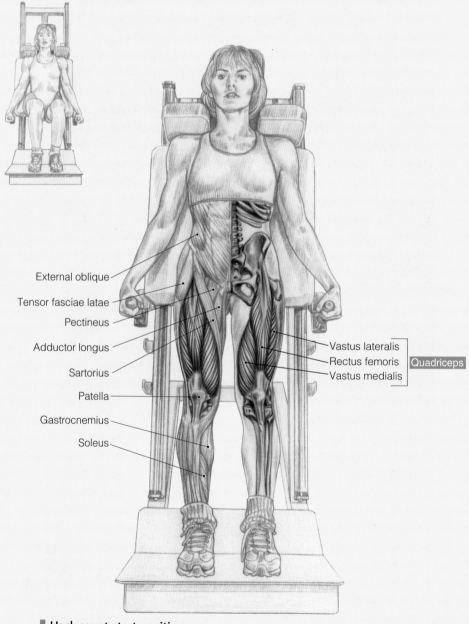

External oblique

Tensor fasciae latae

Pectineus

Adductor longus

Sartorius

Patella

Gastrocnemius

Soleus

Vastus lateralis
Rectus femoris — Quadriceps
Vastus medialis

▌ Hack squat start position

- Squats using a roman chair to block your feet allow you to keep your back straighter than you can with regular squats, but this position will shift the muscular recruitment from the glutes to the quadriceps, which may not be your goal.

▌ Start position

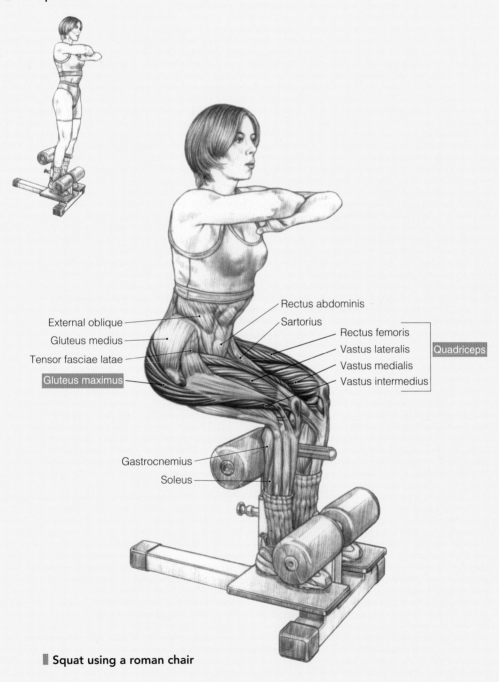

External oblique
Gluteus medius
Tensor fasciae latae
Gluteus maximus

Rectus abdominis
Sartorius
Rectus femoris
Vastus lateralis
Vastus medialis
Vastus intermedius
Quadriceps

Gastrocnemius
Soleus

▌ Squat using a roman chair

LEG PRESS

The leg press belongs in the basic, multiple-joint exercise category because the hip, knee, and ankle joints are mobilized. As a result, the leg press recruits muscles in addition to the quadriceps: the glutes, hamstrings, and calves.

The leg press is considered safer than the squat because it places less pressure on the lower back (which does not mean no pressure). Furthermore, the seat of the leg press machine offers good back support, which limits the risks of an accidental back twist. Also, because the trajectory of the movement is completely guided by the machine, fewer balance problems occur.

There are plenty of versions of the leg press. You can sit or lie in the seat. Also, you can vary the inclination of the machine tremendously, which can make it hard to choose a version. It is best to choose the one that feels the most comfortable (i.e., places the least pressure on your lower back and your knees). Most women prefer sitting to lying. You should also choose based on how you feel your muscles (glutes and quadriceps).

How to Do It

Sit in the machine with your feet about shoulder-width apart on the foot platform. Keeping your back as straight as possible, bend your legs. Do not go all the way down! Stop whenever you feel your buttocks start to lift off the seat. At that moment, push with your thighs to straighten your legs. Once they are almost straight, perform another repetition.

Pro

- Because the movement is guided and the lower back is well supported, the leg press is one of the safest lower-body exercises.

Con

- Some leg presses are poorly designed, and even a very good leg press machine may not suit your morphology.

> **The leg press may seem to be totally safe for the lower back. It is not! Although it is much safer than the squat, your spine will receive a great deal of pressure especially if you use an ample range of motion.**

Tips

- The more you straighten your legs, the more you lose muscular tension. To remedy this problem, avoid fully straightening your legs at the top of the press so that you maintain continuous tension. The exercise becomes much more difficult when you do this because the muscles can no longer rest at the top. You can begin the exercise without straightening your legs. At failure, straighten them a little more so that you can rest somewhat and do a few more repetitions.

Start position

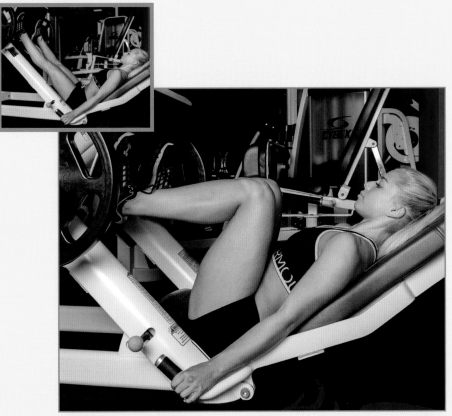

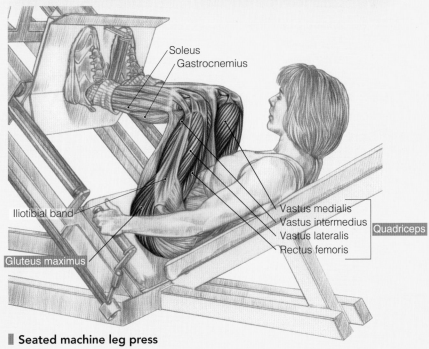

Soleus
Gastrocnemius

Iliotibial band

Gluteus maximus

Vastus medialis
Vastus intermedius
Vastus lateralis
Rectus femoris

Quadriceps

Seated machine leg press

Tips

- The wider your stance or greater your step is, the more your glutes and hamstrings have to work. Leaning your torso forward a little has the same effect.

- Lifting your low back off the seat increases the range of motion of the exercise and enhances the recruitment of your glutes. However, although this may seem like a great idea, it will endanger your lower back. So, we do not recommend it.

- **Warning:** Just as with the squat (see page 78), if you have a recurvatum (hyperextension) at the knee level (you can straighten your legs so far that your knees are pushed backward), *do not* straighten your legs at all because the load can damage your knees in that precarious position. Worse, your legs could bend backward under the load, which would result in very serious injuries.

Variations

- **Varying level of descent:** The lower you go, the more difficult the press becomes because it recruits a growing number of muscle groups. However, the level of descent must take into account not only the muscles you want to focus on but also your morphology. The longer your legs are, particularly your thighs, the more dangerous it is for your lower back and your knees if you go very low. An unfavorable leg-to-torso ratio will result in your having to lift your buttocks off the seat to keep lowering the foot platform, which increases the tension on your spine.

- **Varying foot placement:** You can adopt just about any foot position you wish to better target the muscle group you want. Following are foot placements and the muscles they recruit:

  - **High on the platform:** glutes and hamstrings (spares the knees)
  - **Low on the platform:** quadriceps (this position is tougher on the knees)
  - **Together:** quadriceps
  - **Wide apart:** adductors

Feet high on the platform

Strong use of the glutes and the hamstrings

Feet low on the platform

Strong use of the quadriceps

Feet close together

Strong use of the quadriceps

Feet apart

Strong use of the adductors

The lunge belongs in the basic, multiple-joint exercise category because the hip, knee, and ankle joints are mobilized. As a result, the lunge recruits muscles in addition to the quadriceps: the glutes, hamstrings, and calves.

How to Do It

From a starting position with your feet together and both legs straight, take a step forward with your right leg. At first, go down about 8 to 10 inches (about 20 cm). As you get stronger, you will be able to use a greater range of motion to make the exercise more difficult. Once you reach the bottom position, push back up with the right leg. Don't straighten the right leg completely; keeping a slight bend maintains constant tension in the muscles. After completing a set with the right leg, move on to the left leg with minimal rest.

Beginners can bend the rear leg if they lack flexibility. As you get used to this exercise, little by little, your muscles will get more flexible. You will find the lunges more challenging by gradually keeping the rear leg straighter and straighter.

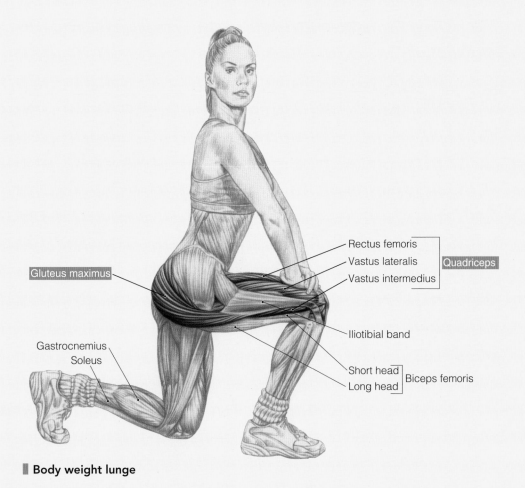

Gluteus maximus

Rectus femoris
Vastus lateralis — Quadriceps
Vastus intermedius

Iliotibial band

Gastrocnemius
Soleus

Short head
Long head — Biceps femoris

▌Body weight lunge

If you are new to lunges or feel that you are going to face balance issues, use one hand to hold something solid, like a wall or chair, for balance. As you get more advanced, placing your hands on your hips will allow you to train your balance as well as your muscles.

Pros

- Lunges are both a muscle builder and an excellent stretching movement.
- If you had to select only one leg exercise, it should be lunges; they recruit the quadriceps, hamstrings, and buttocks.
- Very little equipment is required to perform lunges.
- Body weight lunges will provide very little lower back stress. Even weighted lunges are far safer for the spine than squats.

Con

- Working one leg at a time can be time-consuming.

 The farther or more heavily you step, the more stress your kneecap will receive.

Tips

- Rest your free hand (if you have one) on the muscle you want to isolate (glutes or quadriceps) to better feel the muscle contracting.
- Because the psoas major muscle is stretched during each step, lunges have a tendency to arch the low back. Pay attention to your spinal posture especially if you add extra resistance by holding weights.
- The wider your stance or greater your step is, the more your glutes and hamstrings have to work. Leaning your torso forward a little has the same effect.

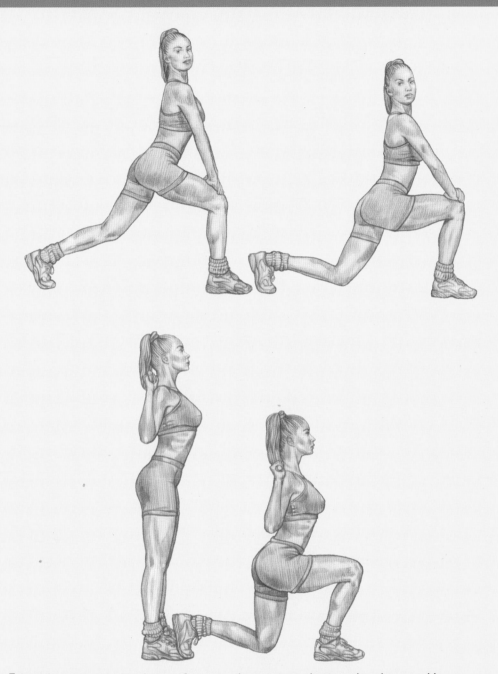

A wide stance (top) or longer first step (bottom) emphasizes the glutes and hamstrings more.

Tip

- A narrower stance or step preferentially targets the quadriceps.

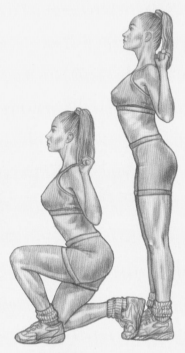

▌ **A narrow stance or first step emphasizes the quadriceps more.**

Variations

- As noted earlier, the first step you take forward determines the range of motion of the exercise. It can be narrow or wide. Begin with a small step to help you master the exercise. To increase the difficulty, take progressively larger steps. You can take a step forward or backward, depending on your preference.
- Alternate legs on every repetition, or do an entire set on one leg and then move to the other leg.
- Stand up completely or rest your foot on the floor and do only a partial movement.
- Add weight by holding a dumbbell in each hand or a bar or staff on your shoulders.

▍Lunge variation with dumbbells

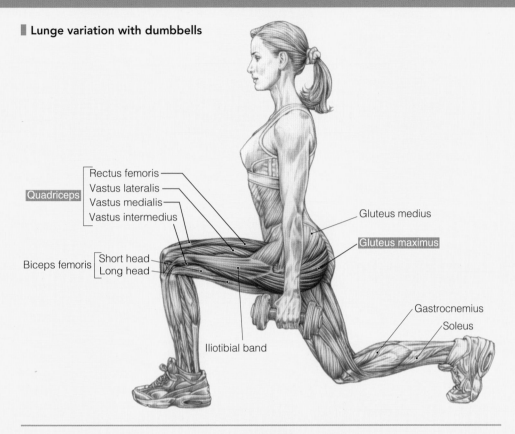

Quadriceps
- Rectus femoris
- Vastus lateralis
- Vastus medialis
- Vastus intermedius

Biceps femoris
- Short head
- Long head

Gluteus medius

Gluteus maximus

Iliotibial band

Gastrocnemius

Soleus

▍Lunge variation with a bar

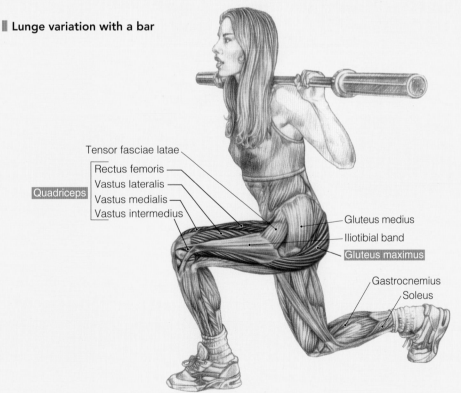

Tensor fasciae latae

Quadriceps
- Rectus femoris
- Vastus lateralis
- Vastus medialis
- Vastus intermedius

Gluteus medius

Iliotibial band

Gluteus maximus

Gastrocnemius

Soleus

Variations

- If you have space, do walking lunges across a room or outdoors. You can also perform walking lunges on a treadmill.
- Instead of doing a forward lunge, do a side lunge. Side lunges are riskier for the knees, but they recruit the adductors more powerfully than regular lunges do.

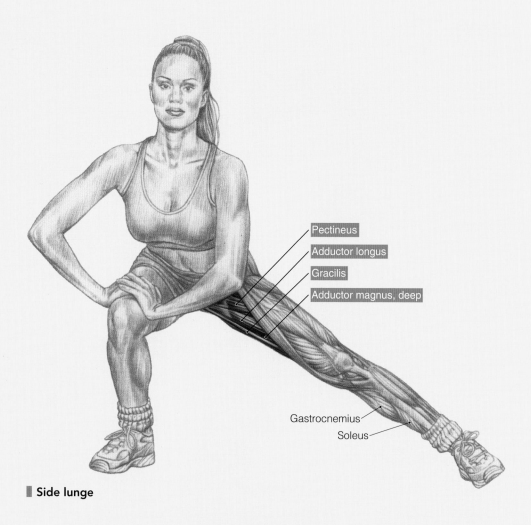

Pectineus
Adductor longus
Gracilis
Adductor magnus, deep

Gastrocnemius
Soleus

▌ **Side lunge**

- You do not have to use extra weights to render the exercise more difficult. By putting the foot of your working leg on a bench, you add resistance on your thigh without putting any additional pressure on your spine.

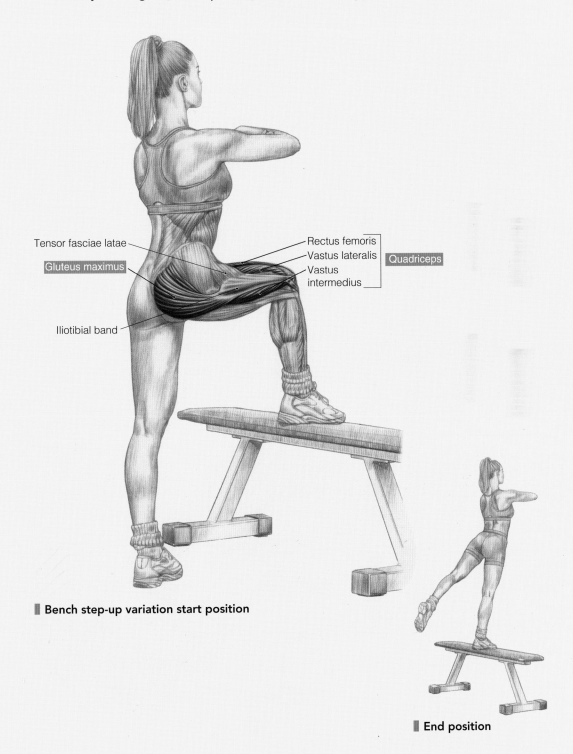

Tensor fasciae latae

Gluteus maximus

Iliotibial band

Rectus femoris

Vastus lateralis

Vastus intermedius

Quadriceps

Bench step-up variation start position

End position

105

LEG EXTENSION

The leg extension belongs in the isolated, single-joint exercise category because only the knee joint is mobilized. As a consequence, the leg extension does not recruit many of the muscle groups surrounding the quadriceps. Leg extensions are often used to warm up the knees at the beginning of a leg workout.

How to Do It

Sit in a leg extension machine and position your feet under the padded frame. Using your quadriceps, straighten your legs. Keep the contracted position for at least one second before bending your legs and repeating the movement.

▌**Machine leg extension**

▌**The movement**

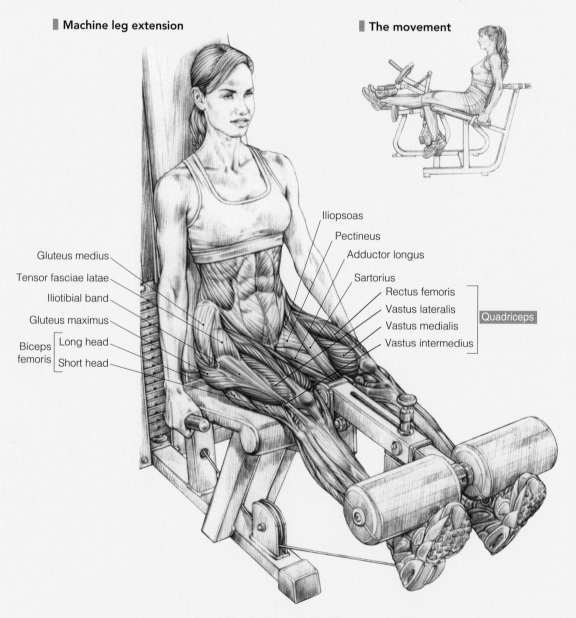

Iliopsoas
Pectineus
Adductor longus
Sartorius
Rectus femoris
Vastus lateralis
Vastus medialis
Vastus intermedius

Quadriceps

Gluteus medius
Tensor fasciae latae
Iliotibial band
Gluteus maximus
Biceps femoris — Long head
Short head

Pro

- Unlike most quadriceps exercises, there is no compression of the spine.

Con

- The leg extension is used to increase the definition of each head of the quadriceps. The glutes are not recruited at all; therefore, if glute development is your main goal, this is not the best exercise for you.

The knee is placed in a precarious position because the quadriceps was designed to contract in concert with the hamstrings to create equal tension on the knees. If your knees are fragile, leg extensions may hurt your joints.

Tips

- Put your hands on your quadriceps to better feel the contraction.
- Don't arch your lower back in an attempt to create a stronger quadriceps contraction.

Variation

If you don't have access to a leg extension machine, you can perform the exercise while sitting, one leg at a time. You can also use a pair of ankle weights for added resistance.

Leg extension variation using a chair

Stand up and bend your right leg behind so you can grab it with your hand. Hold the stretched position for 10 to 20 seconds while breathing normally before moving to the other thigh. Be careful not to arch your lower back excessively.

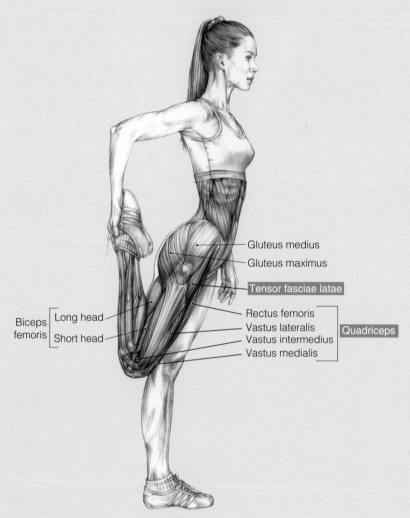

Gluteus medius
Gluteus maximus
Tensor fasciae latae
Rectus femoris
Vastus lateralis
Vastus intermedius
Vastus medialis
Quadriceps

Biceps femoris — Long head — Short head

▍Standing quadriceps stretch

Anatomy and Morphology

The hamstrings (the backs of the thighs) contain a group of four heads:

1. Biceps femoris, short head
2. Biceps femoris, long head
3. Semimembranosus
4. Semitendinosus

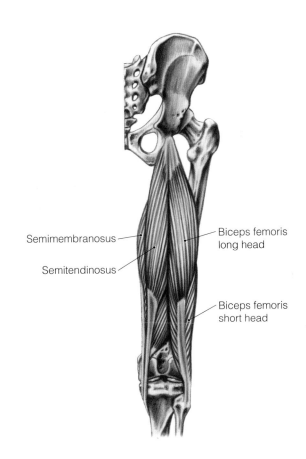

Semimembranosus

Semitendinosus

Biceps femoris
long head

Biceps femoris
short head

The adductors comprise several muscles; following are the major ones:

1. Adductor magnus
2. Adductor longus
3. Adductor minimus

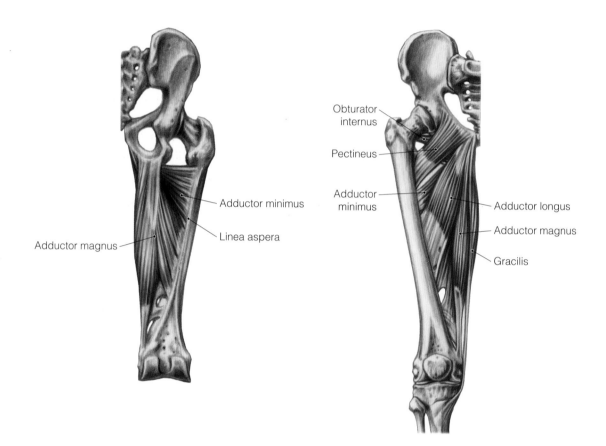

We discuss the adductors along with the hamstrings because the two have a lot in common. Part of the hamstrings serve as adductors, and part of the adductor muscles, which bring the legs together, work alongside the hamstrings in their leg flexor function.

Hamstrings, for the most part, are multiple-joint muscles (one small section is not). The hamstrings are locomotion muscles, but their mode of contraction when we walk or run is unusual because they are almost completely a multi-joint muscle. As we step forward, we contract the hamstrings at the knee while we stretch them at the hip. This stretch accumulates elastic energy that we can use as the leg travels backward. This way, we move our bodies in an economical fashion for long periods.

Despite their key role in walking and running, the hamstrings are often neglected aesthetically, which is a mistake, because they have a key role in shaping the thigh. If you don't walk or run frequently, fat tends to accumulate on the hamstrings, especially at the very top. Weight training as well as cardio workouts on a stepper or treadmill provide a good way to get rid of this fat. Because large fat deposits are common over the upper hamstrings in women, working them in long sets is especially important.

Take-Home Lesson for Women

The hamstrings' placement just below the glutes helps enhance the feminine curvature of the buttocks. Having round buttocks and flat hamstrings would look odd. The hamstrings should be round as well, to accentuate the roundness of the glutes.

The adductors are not muscles you want to make bigger. They just need to be very slightly toned. More important, they should be trained with light weights and high repetitions (no more than 25) to prevent the accumulation of unaesthetic fat deposits on them. Another good reason for using lighter weights is that the adductors are very fragile muscles that are easily overstretched and torn. So, little weights with higher repetitions are perfect for them.

Hamstring Exercises

There are three main categories of exercises for the hamstrings, plus one for the adductors, from which women can benefit:

1. Stiff-leg deadlift
2. Lying leg curl
3. Seated leg curl
4. Thigh adduction

Each category has several versions, which guarantees a great variety of movements and allows you to choose the ones that best suit your anatomy, your goals, and the available equipment.

Before working the hamstrings, you need to protect not only your muscles but also the hip and knee joints and the spine. The goals of the warm-up sequence are to prepare the following muscles for training and reduce the risk of injury:

- Lower back
- Hamstrings
- Knees
- Hips
- Quadriceps
- Calves

Perform 20 to 30 easy repetitions of the following exercises using light weights. Move from one exercise to the next without any rest. If you do not feel that one cycle has warmed you up, feel free to perform a second cycle.

Once you have finished this overall warm-up cycle, move on to your first hamstring exercise using at least one light set to warm up your rear legs before handling heavier weights. If you are already warmed up because you have just finished training your quadriceps or your glutes, there is no need to repeat the entire warm-up sequence. However, you should still do at least one set of a specific hamstring exercise as a warm-up.

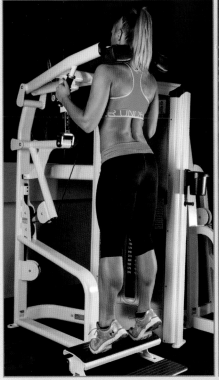

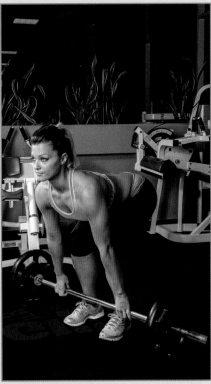

▌ 1. Calf raise (see page 143)   ▌ 2. Classic deadlift (see page 239).

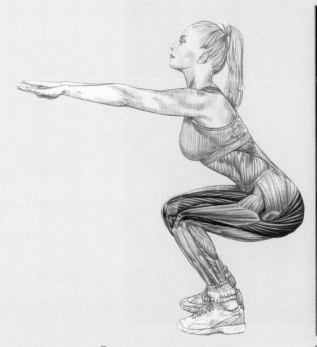

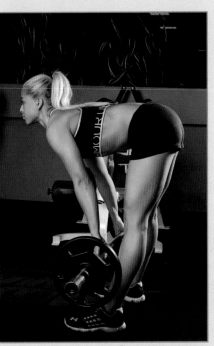

▌ 3. Squat (see page 78)   ▌ 4. Stiff-leg deadlift (see page 114)

The stiff-leg deadlift belongs in the isolated, single-joint exercise category because it mostly mobilizes the hip joint only, even though other joints are placed under extreme tension during the exercise. As a result, the stiff-leg deadlift recruits muscles in addition to the hamstrings: the glutes, lower back, and quadriceps. It differs from the other hamstring exercises in that it provides a strong muscle stretch.

How to Do It

With your feet about shoulder-width apart and your back arched very slightly backward, bend over and lift two dumbbells or a barbell from the floor. Use a natural hand grip with dumbbells—that is, a semi-pronated grip that is somewhere between neutral (thumbs forward) and pronated (thumbs facing each other). Use a pronated grip with a bar.

Stand up using the strength of your hamstrings and your glutes while keeping your legs semistraight. Once you are standing, bend forward without bending your legs to return to your starting position. The weights do not have to touch the floor before you start another repetition.

▌ **Start position**

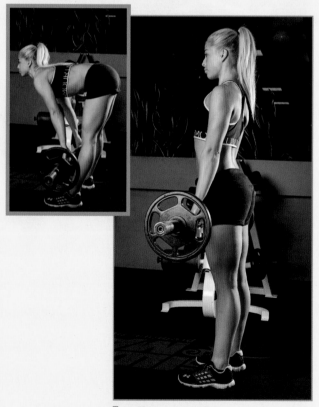

▌ **Stiff-leg deadlift**

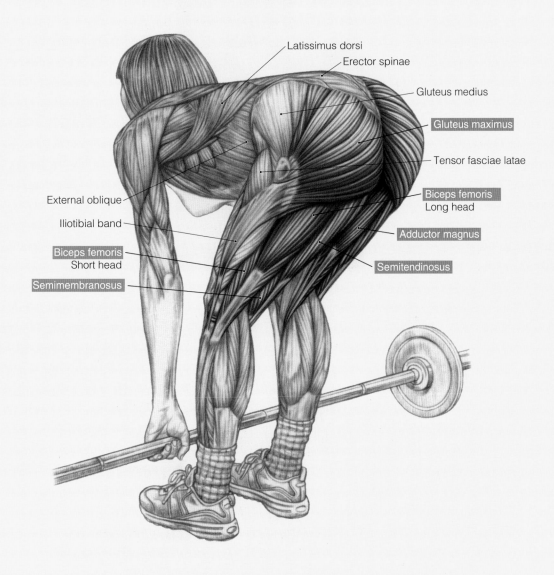

Latissimus dorsi

Erector spinae

Gluteus medius

Gluteus maximus

Tensor fasciae latae

Biceps femoris
Long head

Adductor magnus

Semitendinosus

External oblique

Iliotibial band

Biceps femoris
Short head

Semimembranosus

You may have difficulty at first keeping your legs straight. In that case, do not hesitate to bend them a little. However, keep in mind that bending them too much will reduce the tension on your hamstrings.

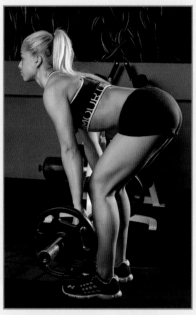

▌ **Deadlift with knees slightly bent**

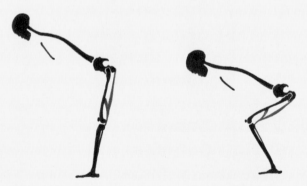

▌ Flexing the knees (right) when bending forward transfers some tension from the hamstrings to the hip and thigh muscles. Keeping the legs straight (left) when you are bending forward stretches the hamstrings, strengthening the contraction.

Pro

- This is the best exercise for working the hamstrings intensely.

Con

- Because it stretches the hamstrings very intensely, this exercise can cause intense soreness that may last a few days.

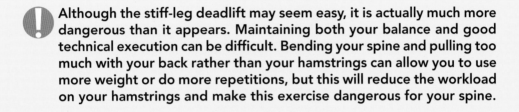

Although the stiff-leg deadlift may seem easy, it is actually much more dangerous than it appears. Maintaining both your balance and good technical execution can be difficult. Bending your spine and pulling too much with your back rather than your hamstrings can allow you to use more weight or do more repetitions, but this will reduce the workload on your hamstrings and make this exercise dangerous for your spine.

Tips

- If you have good flexibility, consider leaning forward with your torso parallel to the ground; then stand up. If this places too much tension on either your spine or your hamstrings, stop the movement short of parallel.

- Do not bring your torso up until it is perpendicular to the floor. By not coming all the way up, you maintain continuous tension in the hamstrings. Only at failure should you come all the way up and rest for a few seconds so that you can perform a few more repetitions.

- When the lumbar muscles tire, maintaining the slight natural arch of the back is difficult. As a result, the spine will start to curve. When this happens, reduce the range of motion so that you can always keep your back straight. The same problem occurs with the good morning variation described next.

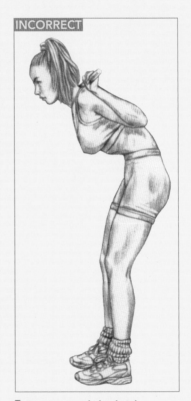

INCORRECT

▌ Don't round the back.

Variation

- Instead of holding the weight with your hands, you can put the bar on your upper back just as you do with squats and bend as in the standard stiff-leg deadlift just described. This variation is called a good morning. This variation will target the lower body more while reducing the involvement of the upper-body muscles, especially the lats, the lower trapezius, and the arms.

▌ Start position

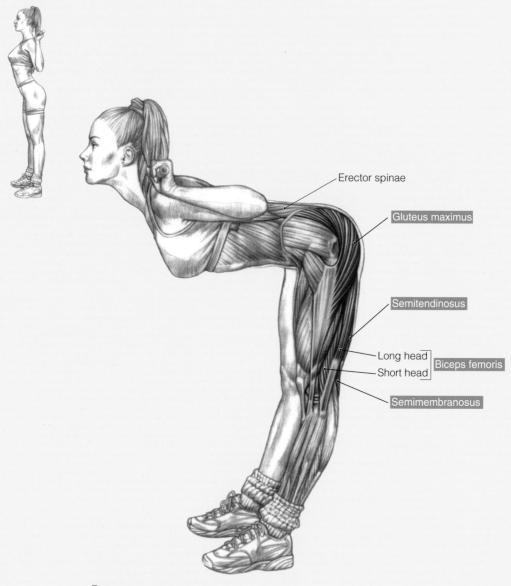

Erector spinae

Gluteus maximus

Semitendinosus

Long head
Short head | Biceps femoris

Semimembranosus

▌ Good morning variation

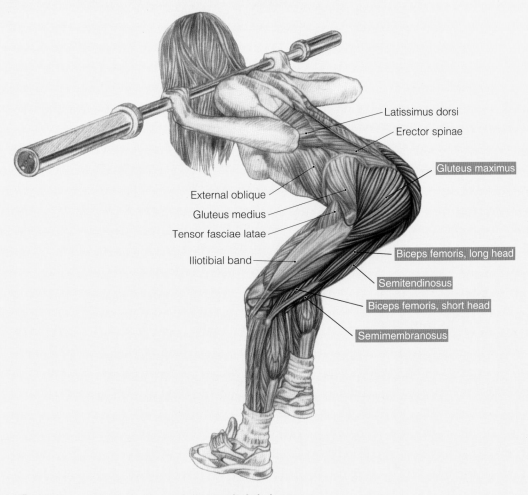

Latissimus dorsi

Erector spinae

Gluteus maximus

External oblique

Gluteus medius

Tensor fasciae latae

Iliotibial band

Biceps femoris, long head

Semitendinosus

Biceps femoris, short head

Semimembranosus

▌Good morning variation with knees slightly bent

FREE WEIGHTS OR MACHINE?

Deadlift machines exist, but they are rare. The main apparatus used for the stiff-leg deadlift is the Smith machine, which provides complete stability and eliminates any balance issues.

The lying leg curl belongs in the isolated, single-joint exercise category because only the knee joints are mobilized. As a result, it recruits only the hamstrings and part of the calves.

How to Do It

Place your ankles beneath the pad of the moving arm of the machine and lie facedown on the machine. Using your hamstrings, bring the pad up to your buttocks. At the top of the movement, hold the contraction for two seconds and bring your feet back toward the floor. Repeat before you have completely straightened your legs.

Pro

- This exercise really isolates the backs of the thighs, which increases your awareness of these hard-to-feel muscles.

Con

- Some women may feel their calves burning long before their hamstrings do because their rear leg isolation is not perfect.

There is a natural tendency to arch the back and lift the glutes during the contraction, which places the spine in a precarious position.

Tips

- Perform this exercise in a slow and controlled manner, not explosively. Do not go all the way back down so that you maintain continuous tension on the muscle.
- Toe position plays an important role in hamstring contraction. Flexing your toes toward your knees recruits the calves as well as the hamstrings, which allows you to handle more weight. By keeping your toes pointed up as much as possible, the involvement of the calf muscles is minimized. This more isolated variation will decrease your strength. In order to best use this unique property, begin leg curls with your toes pointed up. At failure, flex your feet to bring your toes toward your knees. Recruiting the calf muscles in this way will give you more strength to do a few more repetitions.
- Arching your back while bringing your feet up will increase your strength but compress the discs in your lumbar spine. This is why a machine with a bent pad is safer; it supports your spine while preventing you from arching it too much.

Machine Variations

- Some machines offer a very flat surface, whereas others have a bent surface. The bent machines are more comfortable and more effective in working the hamstrings while better preserving the lower back.

▌ Start position

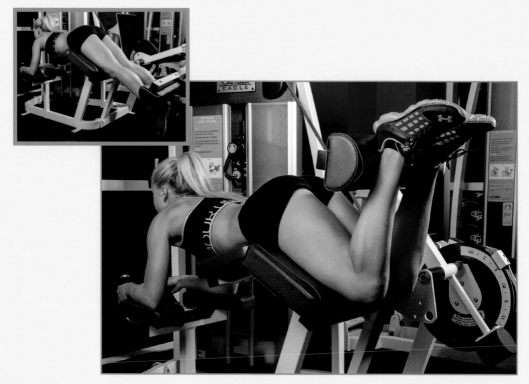

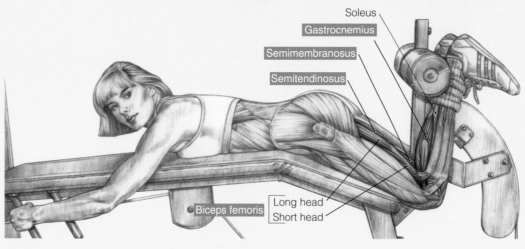

Soleus
Gastrocnemius
Semimembranosus
Semitendinosus

Biceps femoris
Long head
Short head

▌ Lying machine leg curl

Machine Variations

- Some machines have you standing. The standing leg curl is the same as the lying leg curl except that you can train only one leg at a time.

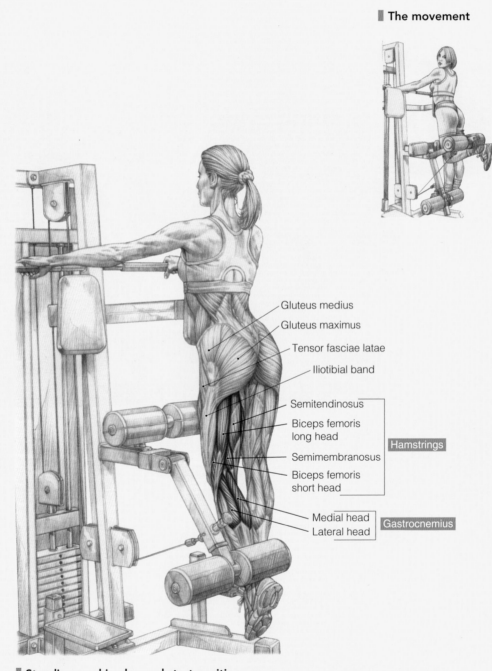

▌ The movement

Gluteus medius

Gluteus maximus

Tensor fasciae latae

Iliotibial band

Semitendinosus

Biceps femoris long head

Hamstrings

Semimembranosus

Biceps femoris short head

Medial head

Lateral head

Gastrocnemius

▌ Standing machine leg curl start position

Body Weight Variations

- If you do not have access to a machine, you can perform leg curls on a bench, standing, or even on the floor. However, your body weight will not provide much resistance.

▎ **Body weight lying leg curl**

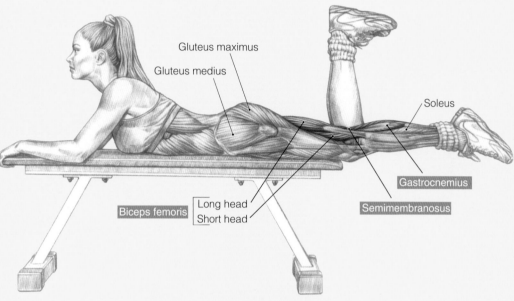

Gluteus maximus

Gluteus medius

Soleus

Biceps femoris

Long head
Short head

Gastrocnemius

Semimembranosus

▎ **Body weight standing leg curl**

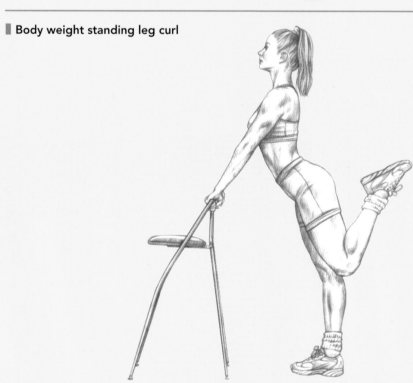

Body Weight Variations

- For a more challenging body weight hamstring curl variation, have a strong partner hold your feet so that you can bend forward as you kneel on a gym mat.

▌ Start position

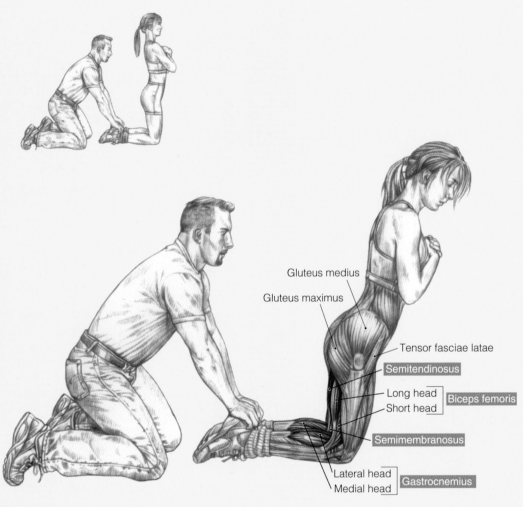

Gluteus medius

Gluteus maximus

Tensor fasciae latae

Semitendinosus

Long head
Short head
Biceps femoris

Semimembranosus

Lateral head
Medial head
Gastrocnemius

▌ Kneeling hamstring curl

Dumbbell Variations

Holding a dumbbell between your feet renders the exercise much more productive. An incline bench is even more effective.

▌Lying leg curl using a dumbbell

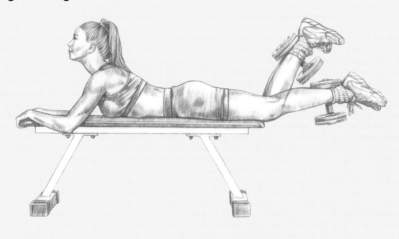

▌Lying leg curl on an incline bench using a dumbbell

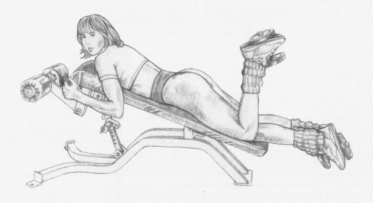

FREE WEIGHTS OR MACHINE?

The lying leg curl can be performed while holding a dumbbell between your feet, or with an elastic band or cable attached to your ankles. However, leg curl machines are safer and easier to use.

125

SEATED LEG CURL

The seated leg curl belongs in the isolated, single-joint exercise category because only the knee joints are mobilized. As a result, it recruits only the hamstrings and part of the calves.

How to Do It

Sit in the machine and place your ankles on top of the pad of the moving arm of the machine. Using your hamstrings, bring the pad down toward your buttocks. At the bottom of the movement, hold the contraction for two seconds and bring your feet back up. Repeat.

Pro

- There is a very powerful contraction of the hamstrings making it the best machine exercise for this muscle.

Con

- With some machines, it is simply not possible to move the torso forward, even slightly.

Start position

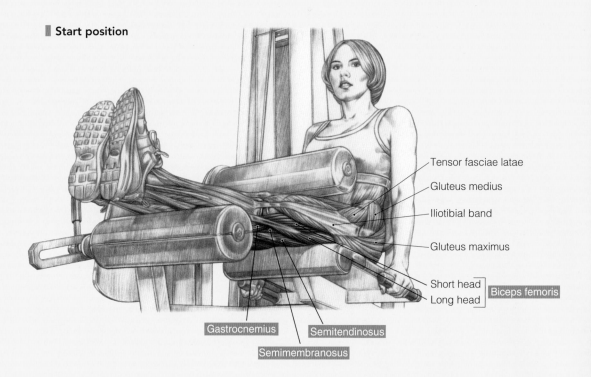

Tensor fasciae latae

Gluteus medius

Iliotibial band

Gluteus maximus

Short head
Long head
Biceps femoris

Gastrocnemius
Semitendinosus
Semimembranosus

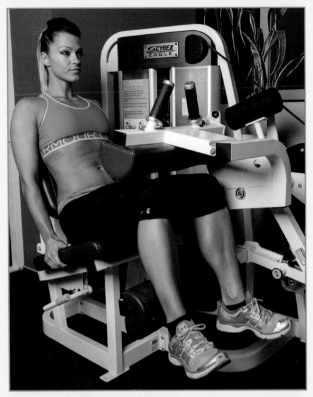

▌ Seated machine leg curl

Sitting firmly with no forward lean may create tension in the spine, causing you to arch your back in an awkward position.

Tips

- Perform this exercise in a slow and controlled manner, not explosively. Do not straighten your legs completely in the stretched position so that you maintain continuous tension in the hamstrings.

- Don't arch your lower back as you contract your hamstrings.

FREE WEIGHTS OR MACHINE?

The seated leg curl can be performed with an elastic band or a cable attached to the ankles. However, leg curl machines are safer and easier to use.

127

Advanced Variation

Even though this is technically an isolation exercise, the seated leg curl is a multiple-joint exercise if you move your torso forward as you bring your legs down.

Notice that when you remain well seated, it is very hard to bring the movement arm of the machine all the way back. As you contract your hamstrings, they become progressively weaker, which forces you to arch your lower back.

This demonstrates the physiological absurdity of staying firmly seated during the entire exercise. By moving your torso forward as your legs move backward, your hamstrings will become progressively stronger instead of weaker as the repetitions go on. Your range of motion in the contracted position will be greater, and there will be no arching of the lower back.

However, be very careful not to lift your legs while you are leaned forward. This could overstretch your hamstring muscles. Bring your torso back as you straighten your legs. When your legs are straight, your back is straight. The farther you bring your legs under you, the more you lean forward. While the legs are bending to 90 degrees, the torso is bending to 45 degrees. The reverse happens when you extend your legs.

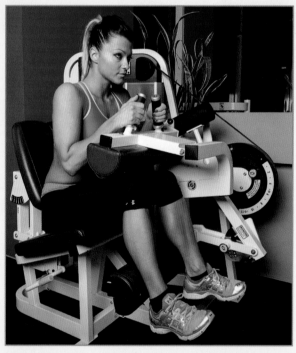

Seated machine leg curl with a forward lean

The thigh adduction belongs to the isolated, single-joint exercise category because only the hip joints are mobilized. As a consequence, the thigh adduction does not recruit much of the muscle groups surrounding the adductors. This is considered a good finishing exercise for the legs because it is relatively easy to perform even when tired as a result of previous thigh movements.

How to Do It

Sit in the machine and place your legs behind the pads of the moving arms of the machine. Using your adductors, squeeze your legs together. When they are as close as possible, hold the contraction for a count of 5 before returning to the starting position.

With most machines, you have to sit. Some newer equipment, however, allows you to perform the movement while standing. Even though standing is not as comfortable as sitting, it is a more efficient way to work the adductors.

▌ Start position

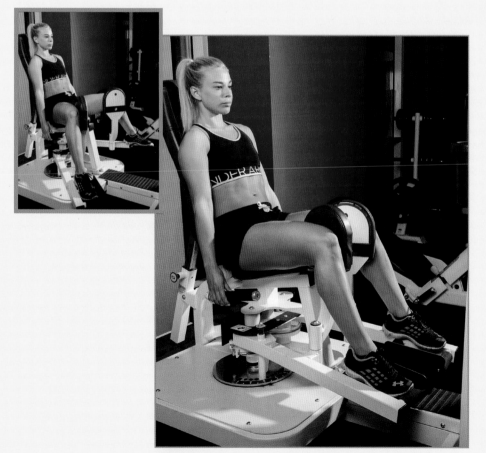

▌ Seated machine thigh adduction

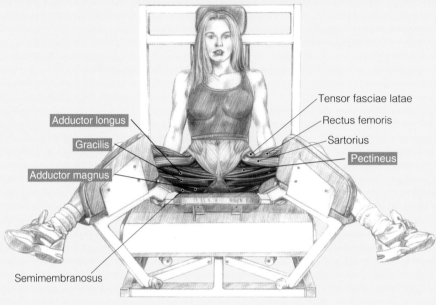

Tensor fasciae latae

Rectus femoris

Sartorius

Adductor longus

Gracilis

Pectineus

Adductor magnus

Semimembranosus

(a)

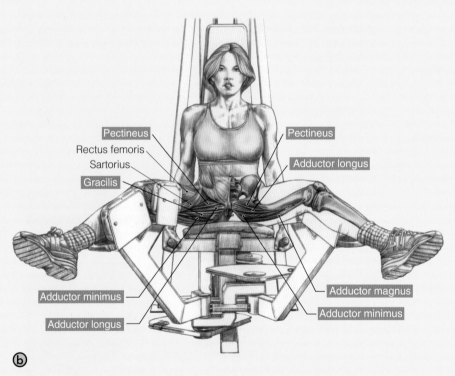

Pectineus

Pectineus

Rectus femoris

Sartorius

Adductor longus

Gracilis

Adductor minimus

Adductor magnus

Adductor minimus

Adductor longus

(b)

▌ Both *(a)* superficial and *(b)* deep adductor muscles are stimulated by adduction exercises.

Pro

- It is hard to really isolate the adductor as well as this exercise does.

Con

- Getting in and out of some machines may prove difficult. Make sure you do not overstretch your adductors when doing so.

 The use of too great a range of motion can tear your adductors.

Tips

- Perform this exercise very slowly over a short range of motion.
- Letting the machine open your legs too wide because you cannot control the weight may overstretch your adductor muscles.

FREE WEIGHTS OR MACHINE?

It is almost impossible to isolate the adductor muscles with free weights. This is a situation in which machines are very handy. If no machine is available, you can substitute with a cable, but adductor machines are easier to master.

Cable Variation

- If you do not have access to a machine, you can use a low cable pulley to work the adductor muscles.

▌ The movement

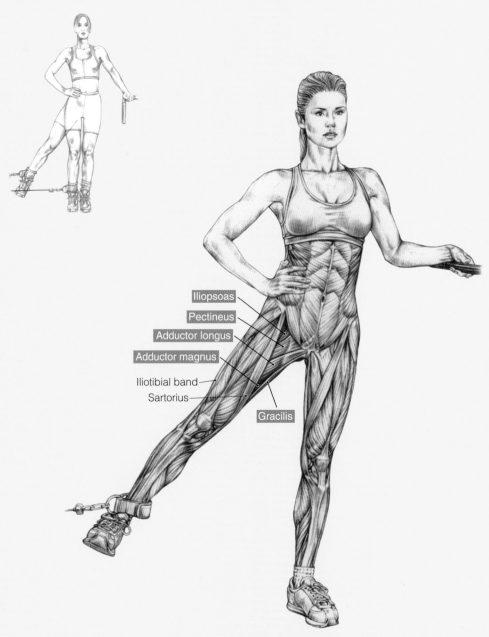

Iliopsoas
Pectineus
Adductor longus
Adductor magnus
Iliotibial band
Sartorius
Gracilis

▌ Standing thigh adduction using a low cable pulley, start position

Body Weight Variations

You can train your adductors at home with body weight exercises or a ball. However, there is little resistance and the range of motion is limited, offering very little prestretch.

- Lie on one side with your bottom leg straight and the other leg bent so the foot is placed outside the knee of the straight leg. Lift the straight leg as high off the floor as possible. Hold the contracted position for one or two seconds before lowering back the leg.
- You can also lie on your side with the bottom leg straight and the other knee on the floor to start the movement.

▌ The movement

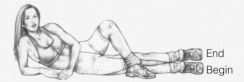

End
Begin

▌ Lying thigh adduction variation with both knees starting on the floor

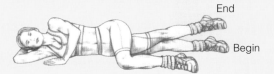

End

Begin

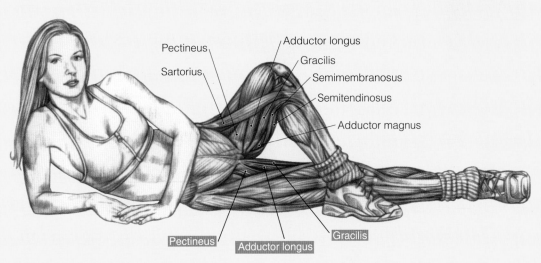

Pectineus
Sartorius

Adductor longus
Gracilis
Semimembranosus
Semitendinosus
Adductor magnus

Pectineus
Adductor longus
Gracilis

▌ Lying thigh adduction start position

Body Weight Variations

- Another option for working the adductors is to perform a squat with a wide stance and the feet pointed out. Remain in the stretched position for one second before moving back up.

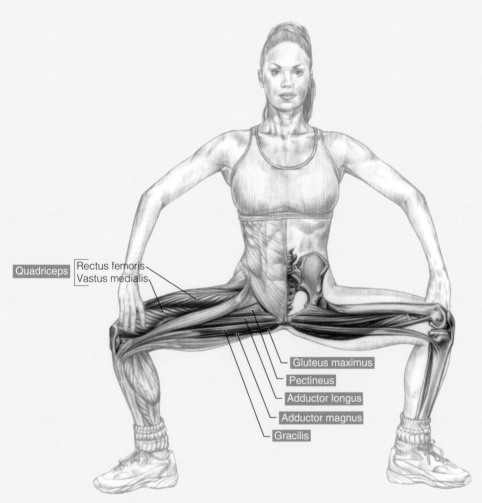

Quadriceps — Rectus femoris / Vastus medialis

Gluteus maximus
Pectineus
Adductor longus
Adductor magnus
Gracilis

▌ Wide squat variation

- Stand with your knees slightly bent with a ball between your legs just above your knees and squeeze your thighs together as hard as possible. You can also perform this ball variation while lying on your back with the ball between your knees. Using a ball will train the adductors in a more isometric way, causing less stretching of the muscles and therefore less soreness in the following days. If you are new to weight training, it is a very good exercise to start with as it will induce less muscular trauma.

▌ Standing thigh adduction using a ball

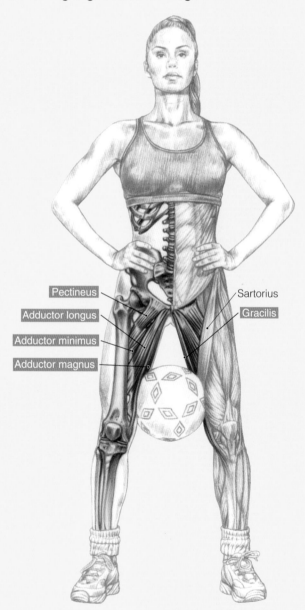

Pectineus

Adductor longus

Adductor minimus

Adductor magnus

Sartorius

Gracilis

▌ Lying thigh adduction using a ball

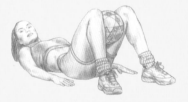

For the following stretches, hold the stretched position for 20 to 30 seconds while breathing normally before moving to the other leg.

- Standing, bend over while grabbing your legs with your hands.

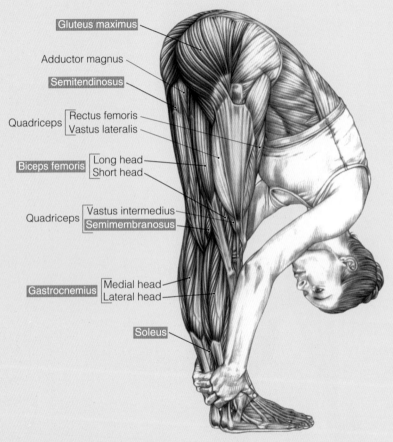

Gluteus maximus

Adductor magnus

Semitendinosus

Quadriceps ⎡ Rectus femoris
         ⎣ Vastus lateralis

Biceps femoris ⎡ Long head
              ⎣ Short head

Quadriceps ⎡ Vastus intermedius
         ⎣ Semimembranosus

Gastrocnemius ⎡ Medial head
             ⎣ Lateral head

Soleus

▍ Bent-over hamstring stretch

- Place one heel on the floor, a chair, or a bench (the higher your foot is, the greater the stretch will be). Straighten the leg and put your hands on the stretched thigh a little above the knee; slowly bend forward. When your hamstring is really stretched, you can bend your standing leg a little to get an even deeper stretch.

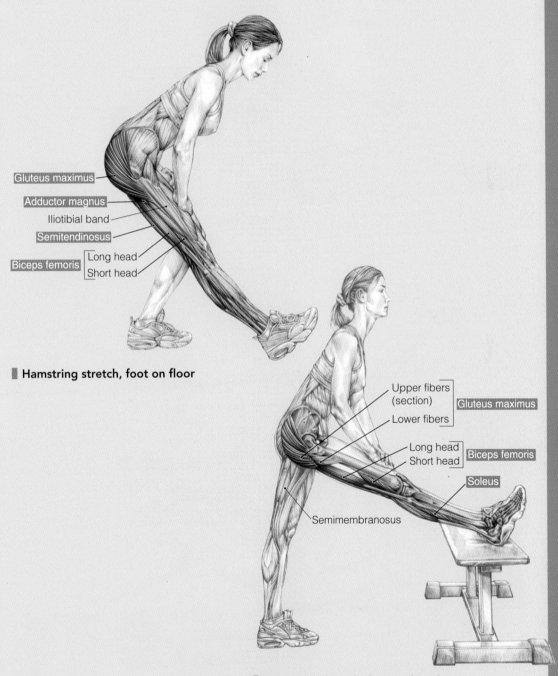

Gluteus maximus

Adductor magnus

Iliotibial band

Semitendinosus

Biceps femoris — Long head / Short head

▌**Hamstring stretch, foot on floor**

Upper fibers (section)

Lower fibers

Gluteus maximus

Long head / Short head

Biceps femoris

Soleus

Semimembranosus

▌**Hamstring stretch, foot on bench**

137

- Lie on the floor and grab one leg with your hands to bring it closer to your torso while bending it (easier version) or keeping it straight (advanced version). The bent-leg version stretches the top of the hamstring but not the lower part near the knee, rendering the movement much easier. It is a good starting exercise for beginners or if you are prone to hamstring strains.

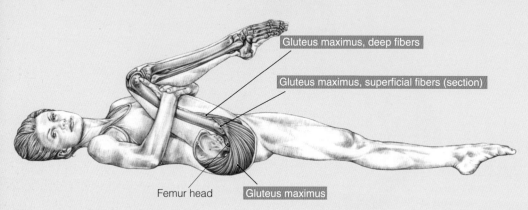

Gluteus maximus, deep fibers

Gluteus maximus, superficial fibers (section)

Femur head · Gluteus maximus

▌ Hamstring stretch with leg bent

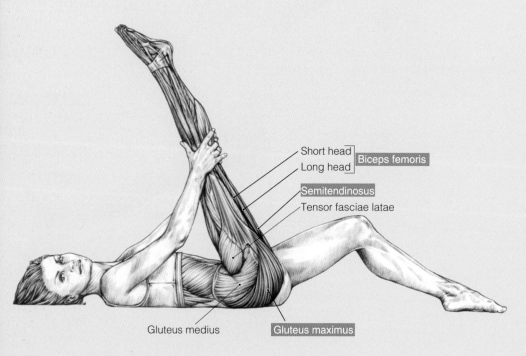

Short head ┐ Biceps femoris
Long head ┘

Semitendinosus

Tensor fasciae latae

Gluteus medius · Gluteus maximus

▌ Hamstring stretch with leg straight

- To stretch the adductors, stand with your legs wider than shoulder-width apart and lunge to the side until the bent thigh is about parallel to the floor.

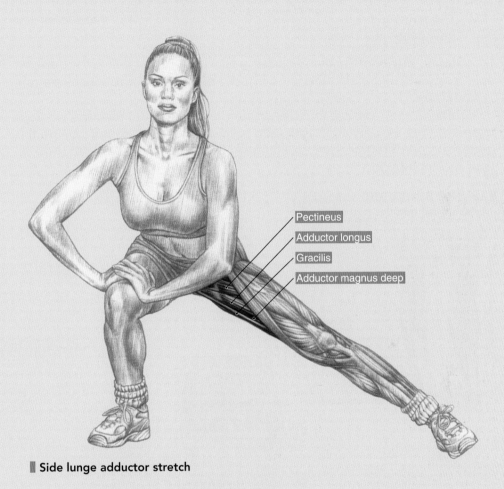

Pectineus

Adductor longus

Gracilis

Adductor magnus deep

▍ Side lunge adductor stretch

Anatomy and Morphology

The calves are composed of two main heads:

1. The gastrocnemius, which provides most of the muscle mass of the calf
2. The soleus, which is covered by, and has much less mass than, the gastrocnemius

There are plenty of smaller muscles around the calves that are indispensable for walking, running, and jumping, but they do not play much of a role aesthetically.

In some women, the calf muscles are very long with short tendons, whereas in others, they are very short with long tendons. No exercise will change this genetically predetermined muscle length. Long muscles are easier to develop than shorter muscles.

▌ **Long calf muscles (left) compared to short calf muscles (right)**

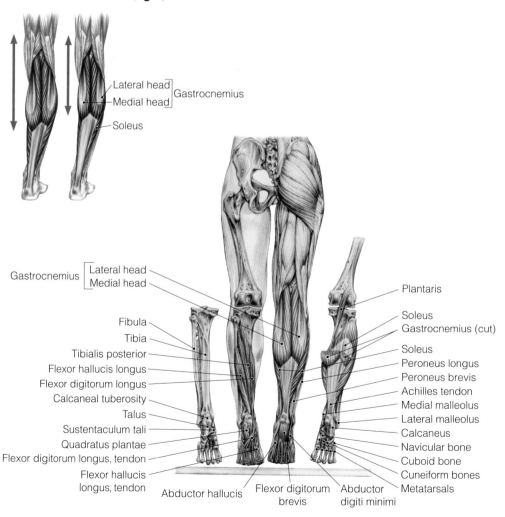

Gastrocnemius
- Lateral head
- Medial head

Soleus

Gastrocnemius
- Lateral head
- Medial head

Fibula
Tibia
Tibialis posterior
Flexor hallucis longus
Flexor digitorum longus
Calcaneal tuberosity
Talus
Sustentaculum tali
Quadratus plantae
Flexor digitorum longus, tendon
Flexor hallucis longus, tendon

Abductor hallucis

Flexor digitorum brevis

Plantaris
Soleus
Gastrocnemius (cut)
Soleus
Peroneus longus
Peroneus brevis
Achilles tendon
Medial malleolus
Lateral malleolus
Calcaneus
Navicular bone
Cuboid bone
Cuneiform bones
Metatarsals

Abductor digiti minimi

The soleus, being a single-joint muscle, is recruited in all the calf raise variations, whether the leg is bent or straight. The gastrocnemius, being a multiple-joint muscle, can only be recruited when the legs are straight or at most only slightly bent.

This is why we recommend that you save time by favoring the calf exercises in which the legs are straight. When the legs are bent at 90 degrees, as with the seated calf raise, the movement isolates the soleus and neglects the gastrocnemius. It is a waste of time for women who are looking to shape their calves.

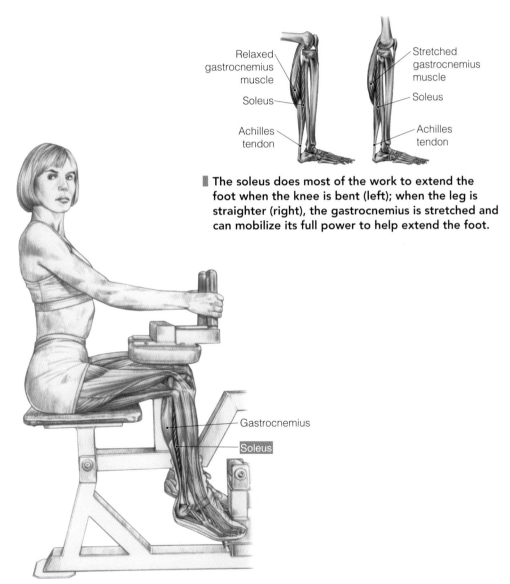

Relaxed gastrocnemius muscle

Soleus

Achilles tendon

Stretched gastrocnemius muscle

Soleus

Achilles tendon

▌ **The soleus does most of the work to extend the foot when the knee is bent (left); when the leg is straighter (right), the gastrocnemius is stretched and can mobilize its full power to help extend the foot.**

Gastrocnemius

Soleus

▌ **The seated calf raise focuses on the soleus to the neglect of the gastrocnemius.**

Take-Home Lesson for Women

The calves are probably one of the most exposed muscle groups (in addition to the arms). Many women aren't seeking large, defined calves but instead are interested in toning these muscles. Therefore, the main goals of calf training should be maintaining proper blood circulation, building some strength, and maintaining good flexibility. As a result, one or two sets of 20 repetitions should be performed at least once a week at the end of leg training. In some cases, cardio training is more than enough for the calves.

If excessive body fat covers your calves, the diet plus cardio training should take care of the problem. In this case, we recommend that you avoid weight training your calves because overweight people tend to naturally build big calves by carrying extra body weight all day.

Nevertheless, stretching the calves is very important especially if you wear heels because they tend to shorten and stiffen the calves' tendons.

Special Importance of the Calves for Seniors

Scientific studies[1] have demonstrated that weak calves rather than weak quadriceps increase the likelihood of tripping-related falls. Therefore, strengthening the calves may directly enhance the well-being of senior citizens. The importance of calf training grows as you get older.

Warm Up the Calves

Because the calves are not a muscle most women want to develop, these aren't the muscles you want to start your workout with. The priority should therefore never be given to calf exercises. In addition, starting your workout with a calf exercise before doing glute, quadriceps, or hamstring exercises can prove dangerous, as it is likely to make your thigh muscles shaky. Doing calf exercises first would ruin your lower-body workout.

Therefore, whenever you train your calves, preferentially after your other leg training, most of the warm-up is already done by the other leg exercises. However, it is still prudent to warm up the Achilles tendon with 1 or 2 light sets of calf raises.

Calf Exercise

Because the seated calf raise neglects the gastrocnemius, the standing straight-leg calf raise is the only exercise from which women who are looking to shape their calves can benefit.

The calf raise belongs in the isolating exercise category because only the ankle joints are mobilized. As a consequence, the calf raise does not recruit many of the muscle groups surrounding the calves except indirectly for stability.

How to Do It

With the balls of your feet (or one foot) on a weight platform or board and your heels hanging off the edge, stretch your calves as much as possible by allowing your heels to hang below the platform. Then, rise up as high as you can onto the balls of your feet. Hold the contracted position for one second; then lower your heels to the floor. If you need to, hold on to a wall to maintain your balance.

▌The movement

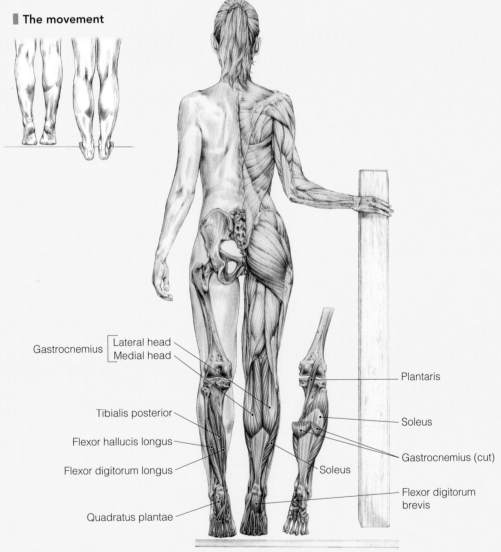

Gastrocnemius [Lateral head
Medial head

Tibialis posterior

Flexor hallucis longus

Flexor digitorum longus

Quadratus plantae

Soleus

Plantaris

Soleus

Gastrocnemius (cut)

Flexor digitorum brevis

▌Standing straight-leg calf raise

143

Pro

- This exercise really isolates the calf muscles.

Con

- If you are doing other leg exercises or cardio training, in many cases doing a separate exercise for the calves isn't necessary.

(!) Make sure there is absolutely no swaying of your body, especially of your spine, during standing calf raises. These movements could be very dangerous for your back, especially as you add resistance to the movement. If you are prone to those undulations, keep your knees slightly bent instead of having your legs as straight as possible.

Tips

- You can perform the calf raise unilaterally to apply the weight of the whole body to one calf. Working one calf at a time provides a better stretch and better contraction of the muscle, which increases the range of motion.

- If you suffer from bad leg circulation, it is very important to train your calves often with very high reps to push back the blood and flush out any excessive water retention. Using your body weight as resistance, perform a set of 50 to 100 reps at home before bedtime or whenever you suffer from lower-body pain.

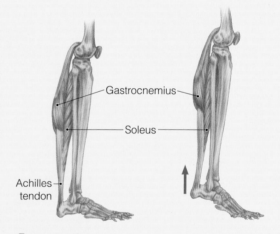

Gastrocnemius

Soleus

Achilles tendon

▐ **Action of the gastrocnemius during the calf raise**

- Many trainers recommend straightening the legs completely to work the gastrocnemius muscles, but the gastrocnemius muscle is actually stronger when the knees are slightly bent because of the more advantageous length–tension relationship.

Dumbbell Variation

- Without any equipment, the calf raise can be performed with your body weight only. If this is too easy, you can do it with only one foot or you can hold a dumbbell in your hand to add extra resistance (or both). Unfortunately, training one leg at a time is time-consuming.

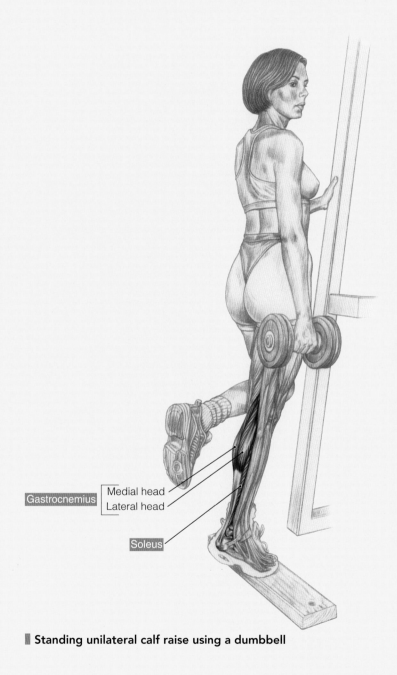

Gastrocnemius | Medial head
Lateral head

Soleus

❚ Standing unilateral calf raise using a dumbbell

Barbell Variation

- Another alternative is to place a long barbell across your shoulders. However, you will not be as stable, and you will not benefit from as big a range of motion.

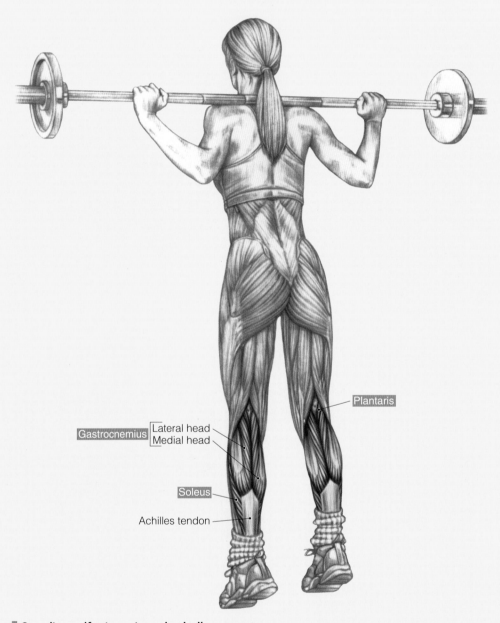

Standing calf raise using a barbell

Machine Variations

- To save time and to have a better handle on the weight, you can use a standing calf raise machine. If you do not have access to such a machine, you can use a Smith machine. Both provide stability, but they put pressure on the lower back.

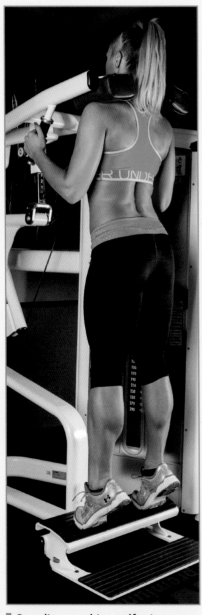

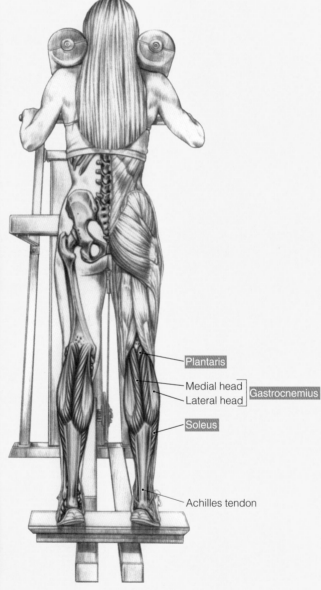

Plantaris

Medial head ⎤
Lateral head ⎦ Gastrocnemius

Soleus

Achilles tendon

▌ Standing machine calf raise

Machine Variations

- A seated or incline leg press machine can be used instead of a calf raise machine. The main advantage of these machines is that they stretch the calves even more because the seated position stretches the calves at the knee level and not at the ankle only. This double stretch is possible because the gastrocnemius is a multiple-joint muscle that can be flexed by the two joints it crosses. These machines also take a lot of pressure off your back. Leg press machines are a great alternative to standing calf raise machines.

- The donkey calf raise allows you to bend your torso to put the calves in the best working position; the gastrocnemius is stretched, which increases its recruitment. In addition, this variation puts less pressure on the lower back, because there is no possible spinal swaying as seen frequently in the standing calf raise. Unfortunately, donkey calf raise machines are rare.

Foot Placement

You may hear recommendations to point your feet out or in while performing the calf raise, but it is better to keep them straight in line with your legs to avoid unnecessary twisting of your knees, especially if you are using weights to increase the muscle work. The calves are strongest when your feet are pointing straight ahead, so turning the feet out or in reduces the calves' strength and also the effectiveness of the exercise. The orientation of your feet will not change the basic shape of your calves.

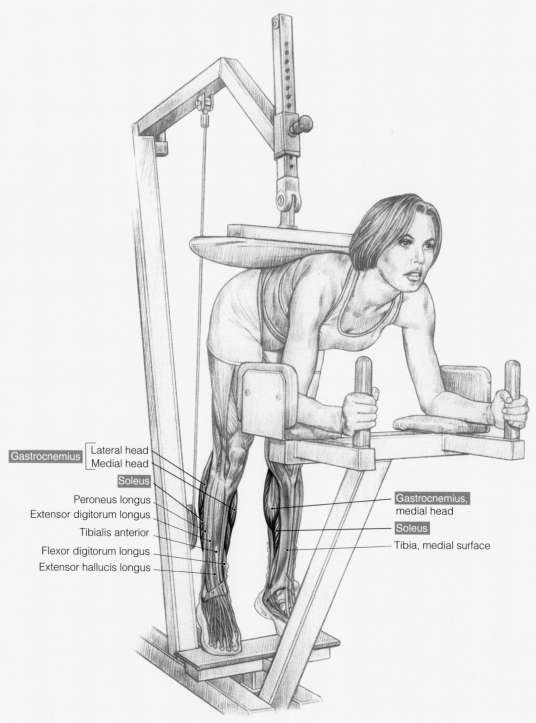

Gastrocnemius — Lateral head
Medial head
Soleus
Peroneus longus
Extensor digitorum longus
Tibialis anterior
Flexor digitorum longus
Extensor hallucis longus

Gastrocnemius, medial head
Soleus
Tibia, medial surface

▌ Machine donkey calf raise

Stretching the calves is very important, especially if you wear heels because they tend to shorten the calves' tendons. On the other hand, if you suffer from calf laxity that is too great (i.e., you twist your ankles very easily), we recommend that you avoid stretching your calves. Instead, you would be better served by shortening your tendons with the calf raise.

You can do calf stretches on one leg or both legs at the same time. The range of the stretch is much greater when you stretch one leg at a time because of the following:

- You are always more flexible during unilateral stretches.
- Your body weight forces the stretch much more when the weight is applied to one leg rather than distributed on both legs.

There are also many angles from which to stretch your calf muscles. As a general rule, do the following while stretching your calves to have the following effects:

- Keep your leg straight to primarily stretch the gastrocnemius muscle.
- Bend your leg to stretch the soleus muscle.
- Twist your ankle to the side to stretch the lateral muscles of the calves.

If your ankles are stiff, stretch your calves thoroughly from all three angles (standing, lunging, and twisting) because each exercise stretches distinct muscles of the calf. These exercises are complementary and in no way redundant.

If you are satisfied with your degree of ankle flexibility, performing the standing and twisting exercises would be enough to maintain it.

- Place the balls of your feet (or one foot) on a weight plate, a board, or a phone book. The higher the object is, the greater the stretch will be. Bend over while keeping your legs straight. Hold the stretching position for 10 to 30 seconds.

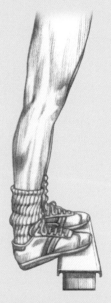

Standing calf stretch

- Do a forward lunge. Placing the ball of the front foot on a weight, a board, or a phone book will accentuate the stretch. The farther forward you place your knee, the more intense the stretch will be. Slowly bring most of your body weight over the foot that you are stretching. Hold the stretching position for 10 to 30 seconds. Lunge backward and repeat with the other leg.

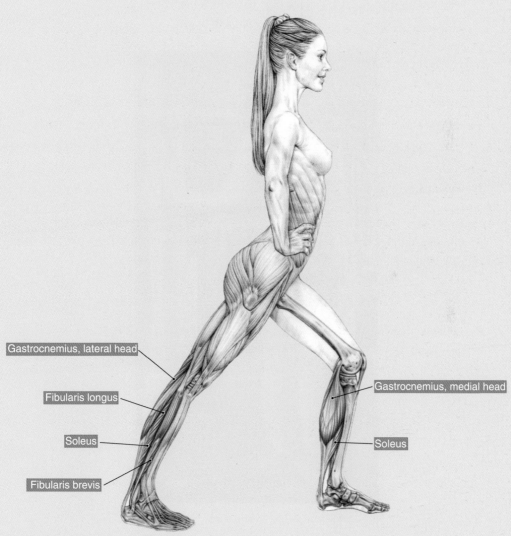

Gastrocnemius, lateral head

Fibularis longus

Soleus

Fibularis brevis

Gastrocnemius, medial head

Soleus

❚ Lunging calf stretch

- This exercise stretches the muscles on the outside of the calves. These are the muscles you strain when you violently twist your ankle. Because the slightest excessive stretch of these muscles will prevent you from walking, it is important to work on flexibility to prevent injuries. Stand with your feet close together and put your weight on your left foot. Roll your right foot as far over to the side as possible. Slowly move your weight over to the right foot. You should do this stretch progressively and slowly so that you do not tear a muscle or a tendon. Once you have stretched the right foot, stretch the left foot.

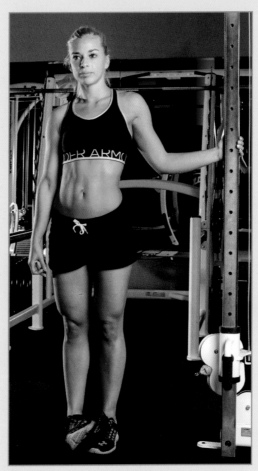

Twisting the ankle to the side

Anatomy and Morphology

The abdominal wall is made up of a very complex mesh of muscles that belong to the group known as the core muscles:

1. The rectus abdominis, commonly called the abs
2. The external obliques, on both sides of the rectus abdominis
3. The internal obliques, under the external obliques
4. The transversus abdominis, under the obliques

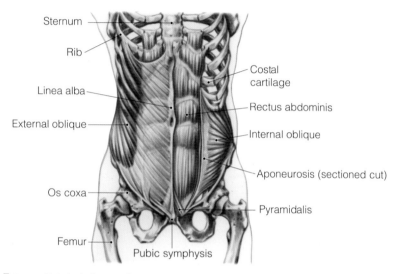

▌ Superficial abdominal muscles

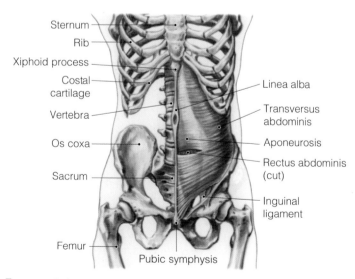

▌ Deep abdominal muscles

153

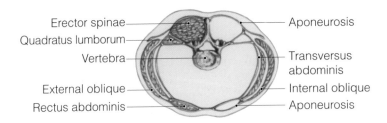

Erector spinae — Aponeurosis
Quadratus lumborum —
Vertebra — Transversus abdominis
External oblique — Internal oblique
Rectus abdominis — Aponeurosis

▎**Cross-section of the core muscles**

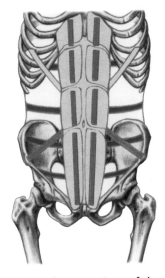

▎**The lines of contractions of the rectus abdominis (red), external obliques (yellow), internal obliques (green), and transversus abdominis (blue)**

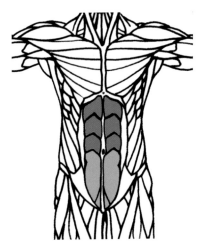

▎**Upper abs (in red) and lower abs (in orange)**

The abdominal muscles contract on both ends. Exercises that lift the torso recruit the upper abdominal muscles mostly; those that lift the lower part of the body recruit the lower abdominal muscles (although, as with the upper abdominal muscles, not exclusively).

The oblique muscles are located on both sides of the abdomen. They support the spine and have a major role in rotating the pelvis.

Unfortunately, the lower abdominal muscles are much more difficult to target and develop than the upper abdominal muscles are. Consider the fact that you can perform leg raises mostly with the strength of your upper abdominal muscles. This makes leg raises harder to execute than crunches.

However, the lower abdominal muscles have the largest role in protecting the spine and keeping off belly fat (which is where fat accumulates most easily). A good abdominal training regimen, therefore, works not only the upper abdominals but also the lower ones.

Take-Home Lesson for Women

Even if you do not carry any extra body fat, you can suffer from a hanging belly because your abs lack muscle tone. By training them regularly for a couple of weeks, you can tighten them up, which will automatically flatten your abdomen.

Even if your belly problems result from an excess of body fat, training your abs will shrink your belly for the same reason even if you do not lose an ounce of fat.

The good news, then, is that the benefits of an abdominal training program manifest in less than a month, providing very rapid gratification. Following the initial tightening of your abdominal muscles, you should get rid of some body fat to continue to shrink your belly and enhance your silhouette.

Women often have one of the following very different goals as far as abs are concerned:

- A very flat abdomen with as little fat as possible
- A little abdomen with abdominal muscles covered by a very thin layer of fat

Some women want to see their abs, whereas others find this sight too manly. Although these goals may seem opposed, they have one thing in common: a well-developed abdominal muscle wall, as opposed to a flabby belly hanging forward because of a lack of muscle tone. So, whatever your goal is, you must work your abdominal muscles hard.

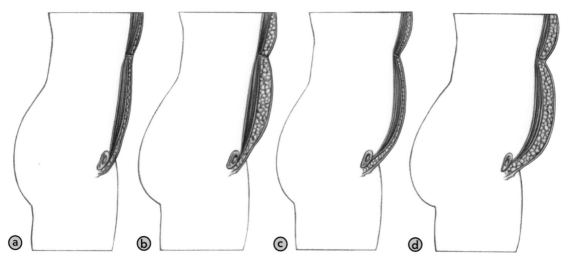

▌ *(a) Normal abdominal wall with toned muscles; (b) normal abdominal wall with toned muscles and a layer of fat; (c) abdominal wall with little tone but no extra fat (the belly hangs out despite the lack of fat); (d) abdominal wall with little tone and a layer of fat (protruding belly).*

Core Muscles and Your Health

When we speak of the abdominal muscles, the first image many associate with them is primarily cosmetic: prominent and well-defined abs are synonymous with a flat belly devoid of unnecessary fat. However, nature has not provided us with abdominal muscles to look pretty.

Our core muscles perform vital functions for locomotion and health. The acquisition of "six-pack abs" is therefore not the only reason to train your core muscles. Following are six good reasons to take care of your abs, in addition to the visual aspect:

1. **Relief of muscle tension.** The lumbar muscles often remain overly contracted during the night, resulting in the spine not regenerating as it should during sleep. The person then wakes feeling tired and with a sore back. A few minutes of ab work before bed can be enough to relax the lower back and release spinal tension.

2. **Protection of the spine.** Along with the back muscles, the abs support the spine. A lack of abdominal tone increases tension in the intervertebral discs, resulting in an increased risk of lumbar degeneration.

3. **Reduced risk of developing diseases such as type 2 diabetes.** Type 2 diabetes develops with age, largely as a result of an excessive accumulation of fat in the abdominal area.

4. **Improved digestive health.** Abdominal work facilitates digestion, preventing bloating and constipation.

5. **Increased athletic performance.** The abs play an important role in all daily physical activities as well as in sports that require fast running or twisting of the core. Studies have shown that athletes with weak abdominal muscles have a higher frequency of side stitches. Strengthening the abdominal wall is a good way to reduce their incidence.[1]

6. **Cardiovascular health.** Circuit training the abs is an excellent cardiorespiratory workout that spares the knees and hips.

Evolution of the Modern Woman

Women have not historically accumulated much fat on their bellies. However, the combination of birth control pills (especially those rich in progesterone) and an excess intake of dietary fat and sugar (e.g., soda, chocolate, bread, pasta, cake) has revolutionized genetics. More and more women now have a gut, like men. In this case, gender equality is not good!

At menopause, the cessation of natural estrogen production upsets the hormonal balance. With lower levels of female hormones, the endocrine system tends to behave in a more masculine way. The result is a disruption of the sites of fat storage: Fat suddenly colonizes women's bellies. For this reason, women must redouble their ab training efforts at the onset of menopause to minimize this reshuffling effect.

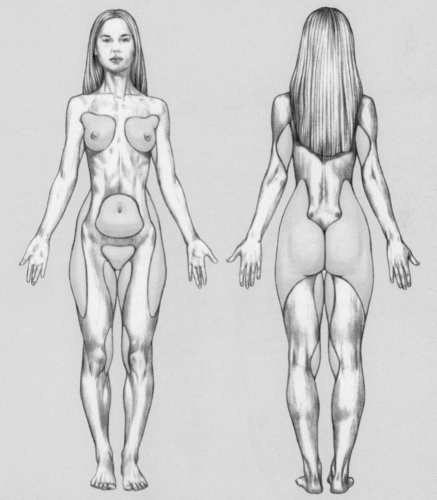

The abdomen and waist are natural fat storage areas in women, but, unlike in men, they should not be major ones.

Spotting Ineffective and Dangerous Abdominal Exercises

The world of fitness is rife with fake abdominal exercises that are not only a waste of time but can also endanger the spine. Fortunately, there is an easy way to tell the good exercises from the bad ones. In a bad exercise, the lower back arches during the contraction; in a good exercise, the back is rounded. Exercises that arch the lumbar spine do not work the abdominal muscles effectively.

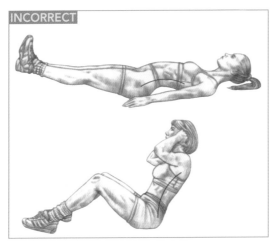

INCORRECT

▌ Bad positions with an arched back

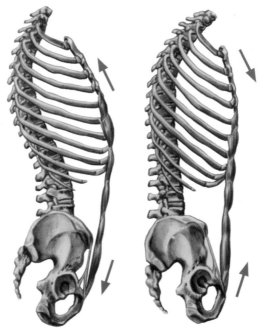

▌ Proper ab contraction (right) brings the rib cage and the pelvis closer to each other. Improper ab contraction (left) brings the rib cage and pelvis farther apart and arches the lower back.

The muscles responsible for movement in ineffective abdominal exercises are the psoas major, iliacus, and rectus femoris. You will know they are involved as soon as an exercise forces you to arch your back. For example, exercises that involve putting your legs in the air for as long as possible and scissors movements while lying down are "back breakers." Because the abdominal muscles are attached to the pelvis and not to the thighs, they cannot make the legs move.

In addition to being dangerous, contraindicated movements are also painful. Because arching the back is dangerous for the lumbar discs, the abdominal muscles intervene to straighten the spine by contracting isometrically (i.e., without moving). Because local blood circulation is blocked during isometric action, the abdominal muscles are deprived of oxygen. Poor circulation also keeps the abdominal muscles from removing lactic acid, resulting in a buildup of large quantities. This movement, which is akin to artificial asphyxiation, causes an intense burning sensation. In addition, it is dangerous and counterproductive to good performance. Keep in mind that isometric contraction does not develop the abdominal muscles or burn fat.

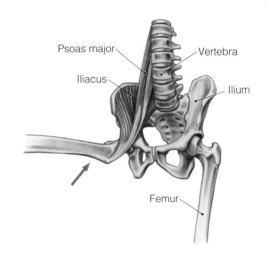

Iliopsoas action during a leg lift

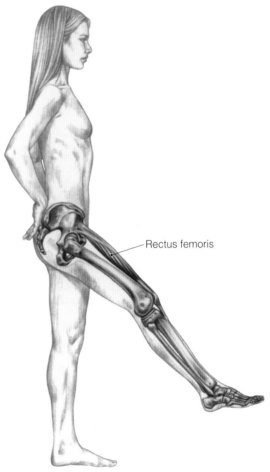

The hip flexors rather than the abs elevate the legs

Enhancing Your Natural Lower Back Curvature

Many consider an enhanced lower back arch much sexier than a flatter lumbar curve. Such a posture enhances the shape of the buttocks and pulls the shoulders back, augmenting the visibility of the breasts, which are many women's goals.

The goals we describe in this book (rounding your buttocks, pulling your shoulders backward, toning your abdomen) are all healthy shaping actions. Enhancing your lower back curvature is easy, but there is a trade-off: more unnecessary tension on the discs of your lower back.

The powerful hip flexors (i.e., the psoas major muscles) tend to accentuate the lumbar arch, sending the intervertebral discs forward. This results in excessive pressure at the back of the lumbar vertebrae, which can lead to back pain or articular deterioration by compression and shearing.

It is up to you to decide whether you want to go this way. If you do, we advise you to do plenty of exercises to enhance the strength of your lower back muscles to reduce the extra pressure you are going to place on your spinal discs.

Whatever your choice is, in this section we describe both ways to perform abdominal exercises in order to do the following:

- Keep your lower back in its naturally aligned position
- Enhance your natural curvature

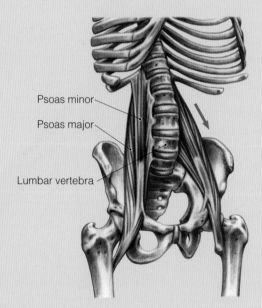

Psoas major muscle action on the curve of the back

Warm Up the Abs

You can either start or finish your workout with ab training. At the end of the training, there is no need for a specific warm-up; just do a very easy first set if you plan to overload your abs with extra weights. If you start your workout with ab work, do at least one light set of crunches before moving to harder exercises.

Abdominal Exercises

There are six main categories of exercises for the abdominal muscles from which women can benefit:

1. Crunch
2. Leg raise
3. Side crunch
4. Twist
5. Static stability
6. Plank

Each category has several versions, which guarantees a great variety of movements and allows you to choose the ones that best suit both your anatomy and your goals.

CRUNCH

The crunch belongs in the isolated, single-joint exercise category. It does not recruit much of the muscle groups surrounding the abs and primarily targets the upper abdominal zone.

How to Do It

Lie on the floor, on a bench, or on a BOSU ball with your legs bent and your feet either flat on the floor or on a bench (putting your feet up on a bench helps prevent the lower back from arching). Place your hands behind or to the sides of your head.

Slowly, without jerking, lift your shoulders and then your upper spine off the floor. Pause for two seconds at the top of the lift while maintaining a strong contraction in your abdominal muscles. Return slowly to the starting position and perform the exercise again, smoothly.

Because emptying the lungs increases the contraction, exhale while contracting your abdominal muscles. Then, breathe in while lowering your torso to the floor. Be sure your head is in line with your spine.

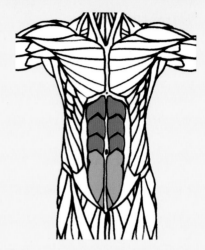

Main areas (in red) and secondary areas (in orange) targeted by the basic crunch

The movement

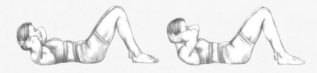

Basic crunch

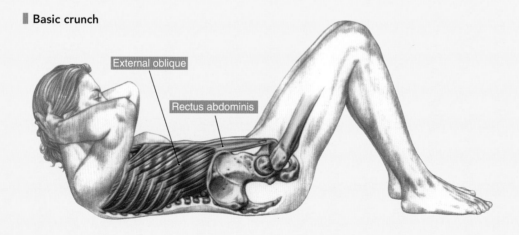

External oblique

Rectus abdominis

Basic crunch, feet elevated

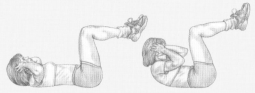

Basic crunch, feet on a bench

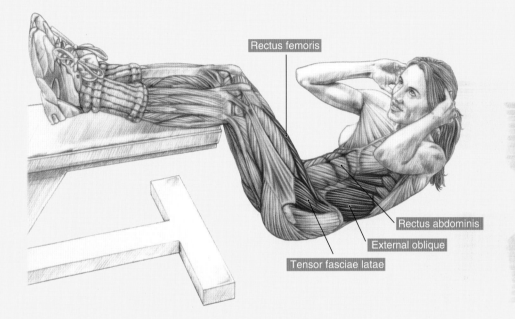

Rectus femoris

Rectus abdominis

External oblique

Tensor fasciae latae

Pro

- The crunch is a simple exercise that targets the abdominal muscles while being easy on the spine.

Con

- The crunch is not an exercise that stimulates the muscles over a great range of motion. Instead, it produces a contraction over a rather small range (about 6 inches, or 15 cm). So, it is of the utmost importance to squeeze the abs as hard as possible during each repetition to make up for this limited motion.

If you pull powerfully with your hands while they are behind your head to get up more easily, you could pinch your cervical spine.

Tips

- You may be tempted to try to increase your range of motion by lifting your entire torso off the floor. This is no longer a crunch, but a sit-up. In a sit-up, the abdominal work is secondary and tension is greater in your lower back. A BOSU ball or a curved bench can help you increase your range of motion in a crunch, thereby enhancing the difficulty of the movement while providing extra support for your lower back. We will show some sit-up variations in the following pages, but be aware of the danger to the spine and consider doing a crunch in situations where a sit-up is shown.

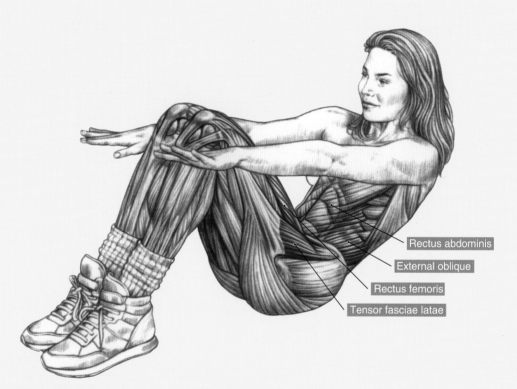

Rectus abdominis

External oblique

Rectus femoris

Tensor fasciae latae

▌ Extending your arms makes the crunch easier.

- Where you place your hands determines the difficulty of the crunch. The exercise is harder when your hands are behind your head, easier with your hands crossed on your chest, and easier still when you stretch your arms forward along your body. Consider this combination: Begin with your arms behind your head, and when you can't do any more repetitions that way, stretch your arms out in front so that you can do a few more.

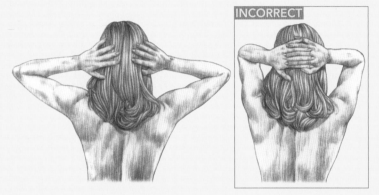

▌ Proper hand position, safe for the neck (left); wrong hand position, unsafe for the neck (right).

- Use a weight plate to increase the resistance. Place it either behind your head or on your chest. Note that a plate provides far greater resistance when placed behind your head rather than on your upper chest.

- Don't tilt your head up to look at the ceiling during crunches. With your head up, you are likely to arch your back. During abdominal exercises, keep your head tilted forward to keep your eyes on your abdomen, but don't tilt so far forward that you strain your neck.

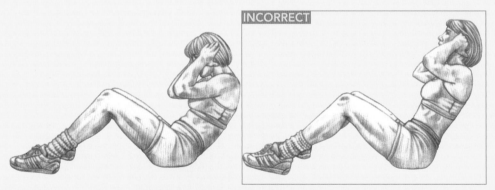

▌ Proper head position (left); incorrect head position (right).

Feet-Stabilized Variations

- Performing a crunch while stabilizing your feet (typically on a wall or by a partner) will enhance your lower back curvature but also puts pressure on your spinal discs. One study showed that whenever crunches or sit-ups were performed with the feet restrained, the rectus femoris was recruited much more powerfully than it was when the feet were unrestrained. The hip flexor muscles come into play far more powerfully when the feet are blocked.[2]

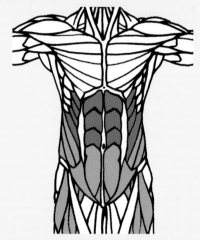

Main areas (in red) and secondary areas (in orange) targeted by the crunch when the feet are stabilized

Sit-up with partner holding the feet

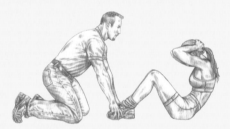

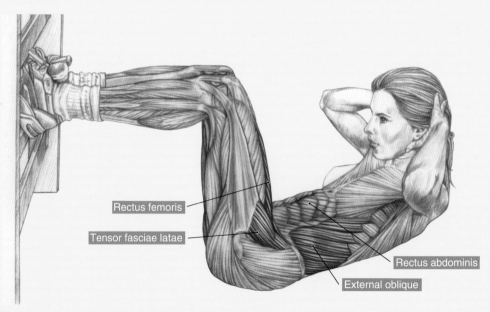

Rectus femoris

Tensor fasciae latae

Rectus abdominis

External oblique

Crunch with feet stabilized on a wall

- If you use an incline bench instead of the floor to increase the difficulty of the exercise, you will have to block your feet to stabilize your body. The higher the inclination of the bench is, the more resistance the abs will have to overcome to raise your torso.

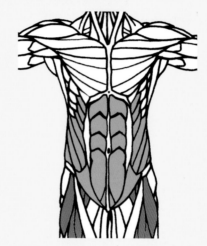

Main areas (in red) and secondary areas (in orange) targeted by the crunch or sit-up on an incline bench

The steeper the incline, the greater the resistance

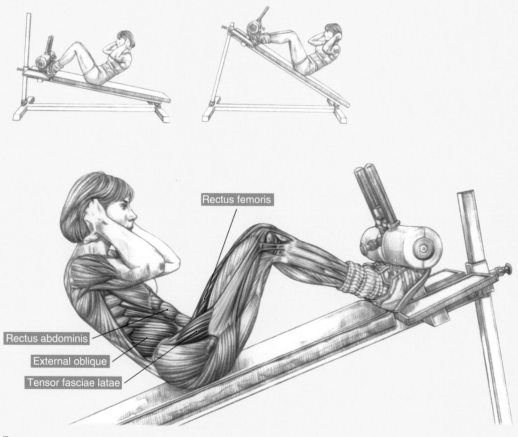

Rectus femoris

Rectus abdominis

External oblique

Tensor fasciae latae

Sit-up on an incline bench

167

Oblique Variations

- To better target the oblique muscles with the crunch, you can rotate your torso to the side instead of coming straight up. As mentioned earlier, the exercise is easier when you stretch your arms along your body and harder when you place both hands behind your head. It is also easier with your feet on the floor instead of raised in the air. To work your left side, gently move your right hand or elbow toward your left knee using your abdominal muscles. Do not try to touch your knee with your elbow; the movement generally stops halfway. Hold the

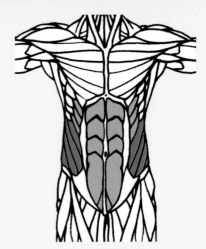

Main areas (in red) and secondary areas (in orange) targeted by the oblique crunch

contracted position for two seconds before lowering. To maintain continuous tension in the abdominal muscles, don't come all the way back down to the start position with your head resting on the floor between reps; keep your shoulders off the floor slightly. Once you have finished on the left side, repeat the exercise on the right.

- Instead of keeping your legs still, you can bring one of them toward your torso in sync with your shoulder rotations in a variation often called a bicycle crunch because of the pedaling motion of the legs. This advanced variation is more difficult to perform because of the more intense oblique contraction it produces.

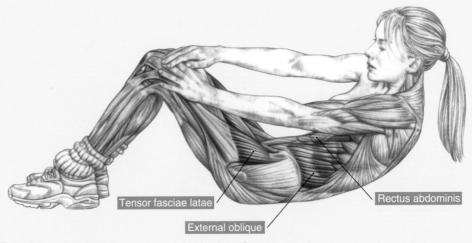

Tensor fasciae latae

External oblique

Rectus abdominis

Oblique crunch with arms stretched out in front (easier)

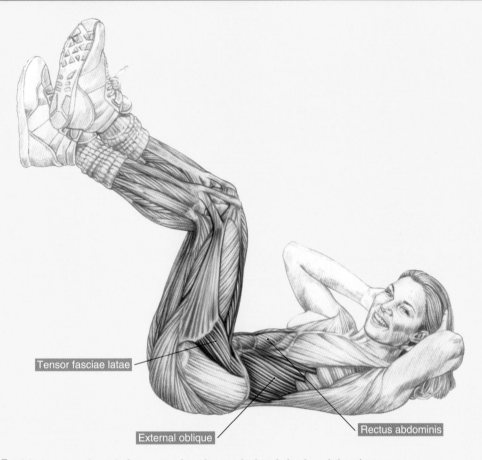

Tensor fasciae latae

External oblique

Rectus abdominis

▌ **Oblique crunch with feet raised and arms behind the head (harder)**

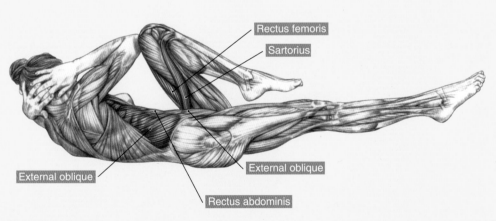

Rectus femoris

Sartorius

External oblique

External oblique

Rectus abdominis

▌ **Oblique bicycle crunch**

Machine Variations

- Abdominal machines are plentiful. Unfortunately, many are not well designed. If you find one that allows you to contract your abs well, use it. But if it feels weird, especially at the lower back level, you are better off with crunches. A good machine lets you choose the precise level of resistance to place on your abs. Crunches might be too hard for a beginner and way too light for an advanced trainer. Machines accommodate everybody as far as resistance is concerned.

- If you do not have access to an ab machine, you can use a high pulley to modulate resistance. An ab machine or high pulley can provide a welcome break if you grow tired of repeating the classic body weight crunch.

- Some home ab devices, such as the ab roller, are well designed and can replace machines.

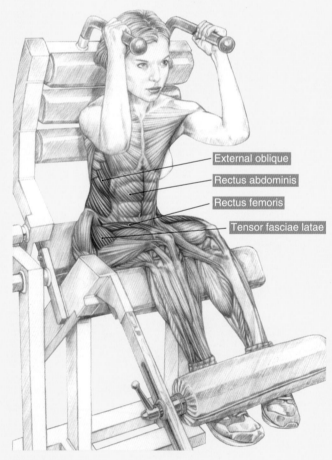

External oblique
Rectus abdominis
Rectus femoris
Tensor fasciae latae

▌ Machine crunch

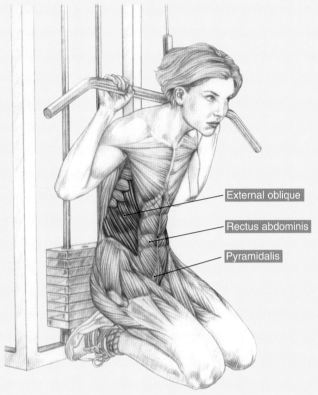

External oblique

Rectus abdominis

Pyramidalis

■ **High-pulley crunch**

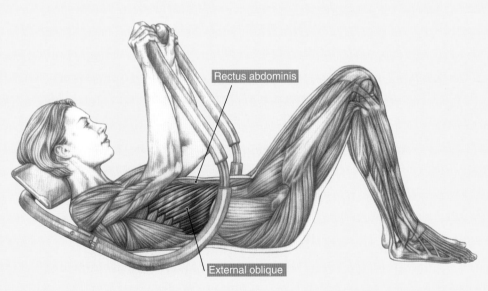

Rectus abdominis

External oblique

■ **Crunch using an ab roller**

LEG RAISE

Leg raises do not all belong to the same exercise category. Those in which your legs remain straight belong in the isolated, single-joint exercise category. Those in which you bend your legs belong in the basic, multiple-joint exercise category. Leg raises recruit the abs as well as the hip flexors. When performed properly, they target the entire abdominal wall but emphasize the lower abdominal area.

How to Do It

Leg raises can be performed while lying on the floor (the easiest version) or seated (harder) or while hanging from a pull-up bar (the hardest variation).

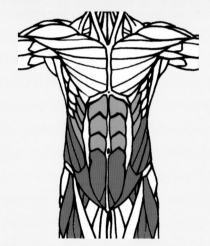

❚ Main areas (in red) and secondary areas (in orange) targeted by the leg raise

- **Lying leg raise:** Lying on the floor with your arms at your sides and your legs bent to 90 degrees, lift your buttocks and then your lower back. Roll slowly and stop when you feel your upper back starting to come off the floor. Imagine touching your lower abdominal muscles to your pectoralis muscles. Although they will not actually touch, visualizing this will help you achieve the correct movement. Pause for at least two seconds at the top of the raise with your abdominal muscles strongly contracted. Return slowly to the starting position and stop before your buttocks touch the floor to maintain continuous tension. Keep your head straight on the floor during this exercise, taking care not to move your neck.

  It is possible to do leg raises that move the legs off the floor very little, but we do not believe that these variations are very effective to firm up your abs.

- **Seated leg raise:** Sit on the edge of a bench with your arms at your sides, holding on to the bench so that you remain perfectly stable. While keeping your legs bent to 90 degrees, bring your lower abdominal muscles up so that they push on the upper part of your abs by rounding your back rather than lifting your legs. The total range of motion is only a few inches or centimeters. Pause for at least two seconds in the upper position while deeply contracting your abdominal muscles. Return slowly to the starting position and repeat.

  The main problem with this variation is that it is harder to roll the abdominal muscles from low to high. The weight placed on the lower back interferes with the mobility of the spine. This exercise is difficult to do sitting down because, if you cannot roll well, muscles other than the abdominals will do the majority of the work.

- **Hanging leg raise:** To make the leg raise harder, you can perform it while hanging from a pull-up bar. Hang on to the bar with pronated hands (thumbs facing each other) about shoulder-width apart. Bring your legs to 90 degrees in relation to your torso so that your thighs are parallel to the floor. You can keep your legs straight (this makes the exercise a lot more difficult) or bring your calves under your thighs (this makes the exercise easier). An advanced combination consists of beginning with the legs straight and, at failure, bending the legs so that you can do a few more repetitions.

  Using your lower abdominal muscles, move your pelvis up while bringing your knees up toward your chest. Lift your pelvis as high as possible while rolling yourself up as much as you can. Hold the position for one second before lowering your pelvis. Be careful not to lower your legs past the point where the thighs are parallel to the floor.

  The hardest thing about this variation when you first try it is to keep your body from swinging too much. As you train more, you will learn to stabilize yourself naturally. Alternatively, specially designed ab benches or chairs provide back support to stabilize your body while hanging.

Pro

- The lower abdominals are the most difficult muscles to work. The leg raise is the best exercise for learning how to work them.

Con

- This exercise is easier done poorly than it is done well. If you feel a pulling sensation in your lower spine, you are performing the exercise incorrectly. Mastering this exercise to the point that you are contracting the lower part of your abdominal muscles properly takes time.

Using your hip flexor muscles too much can place shear stress on your spinal discs, which might trigger pain if they are already damaged.

Tip

- Arching your lower back works the wrong muscles and pinches the lumbar discs. The goal of this exercise is not so much lifting the legs, but lifting the hips, which lifts the thighs.

LEG RAISE

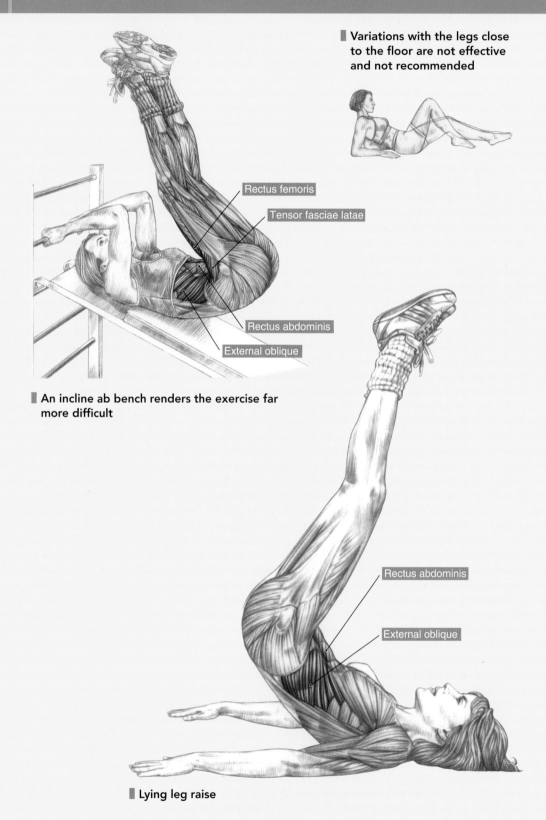

Variations with the legs close
to the floor are not effective
and not recommended

Rectus femoris

Tensor fasciae latae

Rectus abdominis

External oblique

An incline ab bench renders the exercise far
more difficult

Rectus abdominis

External oblique

Lying leg raise

▮ The movement

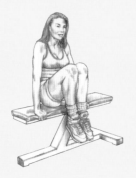

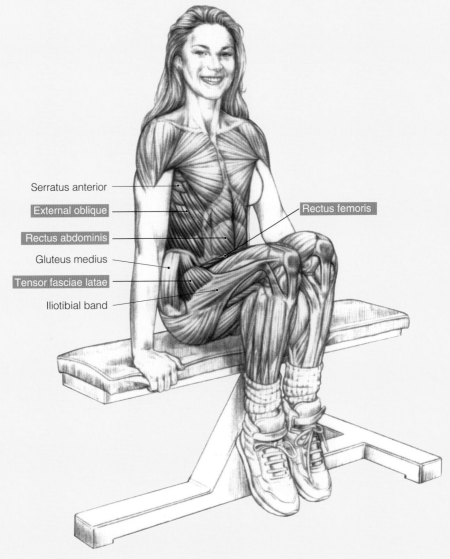

Serratus anterior

External oblique

Rectus abdominis

Gluteus medius

Tensor fasciae latae

Iliotibial band

Rectus femoris

▮ Seated leg raise start position

▌ Rotate laterally to target the obliques more

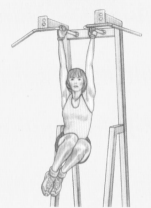

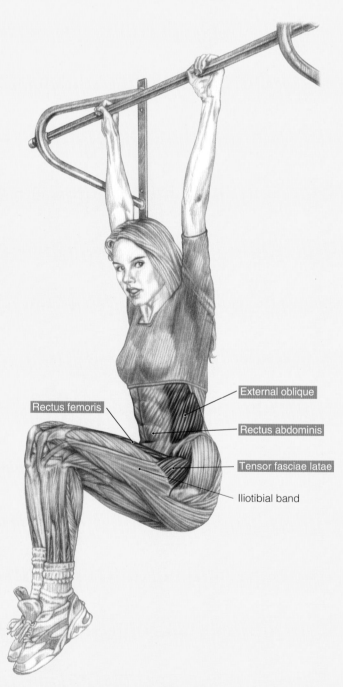

Rectus femoris

External oblique

Rectus abdominis

Tensor fasciae latae

Iliotibial band

▌ Hanging leg raise with a pull-up bar

❚ The movement

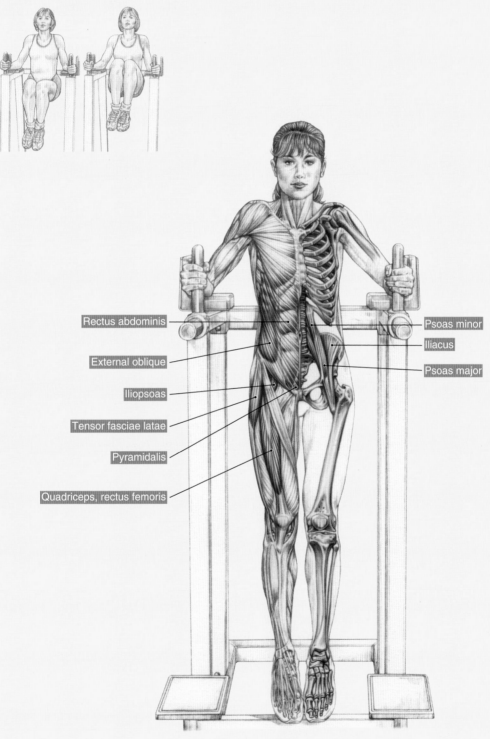

Rectus abdominis

External oblique

Iliopsoas

Tensor fasciae latae

Pyramidalis

Quadriceps, rectus femoris

Psoas minor

Iliacus

Psoas major

❚ Hanging leg raise with an ab chair, start position

The side crunch belongs in the isolated, single-joint exercise category. It does not recruit much of the muscle groups surrounding the obliques and the rectus abdominis.

The side crunch is different from the oblique crunch variation described earlier in that you lie on your side rather than on your back. This exercise isolates the obliques more than the oblique crunch does, which targets both the rectus abdominis and the obliques.

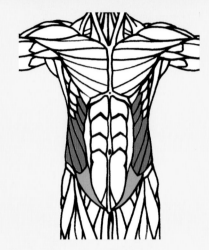

▌ **Main areas (in red) and secondary areas (in orange) targeted by the side crunch.**

How to Do It

Lie on your left side on the floor. Put your right hand behind your head to support it. Using your obliques, bring your right elbow toward your right hip. Your left shoulder will come off the floor about an inch (2.5 cm) or so. Hold the position for one to two seconds before lowering your torso. Bring your left shoulder to the floor, but not your head, so that you can maintain a continuous tension in your obliques. Once you have finished a set on your left side, move immediately to your right side.

Pros

- This is the best exercise for working the obliques.
- You will feel your muscles working immediately if you perform it correctly.

Con

- Using heavy weights with side crunches increases muscle size, but large obliques and a bigger waist are not what you are looking for. Unless you are involved in a strength sport, do not use too heavy a weight when working your obliques. Light weights and long sets will help you eliminate the fat that easily accumulates in this area.

🛈 **Arching your lower back will work the wrong muscles and pinch the lumbar discs. Avoid engaging in jerky head movements to help you do a few more repetitions; doing so will risk injury to your cervical spine.**

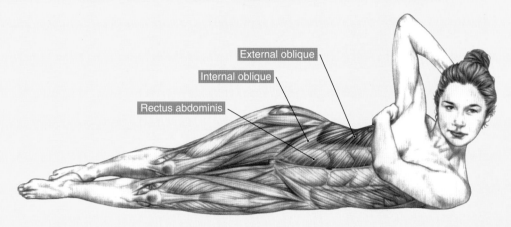

External oblique

Internal oblique

Rectus abdominis

▌ Side crunch

Tips

- Rotate your torso slightly from back to front while contracting your obliques. This exercise is not meant to be performed in a straight line.
- Place your left hand on your obliques so that you can better feel the muscles working.
- Do not begin your ab routine with the side crunch. It is better to end your abdominal workout with the obliques rather than starting with them because your priority should be to work the rectus abdominis.

Variations

- Where you place your free hand determines the degree of resistance during this exercise. The position described here (i.e., your hand behind your head) is an intermediate position. To increase the resistance, extend your arm away from your body and next to your head. To reduce the resistance, extend your arm toward your thighs, parallel to your body.

  Consider using a descending set strategy. Begin the exercise with your arm straight up by your head, and when you can't perform any more repetitions that way, place your hand behind your head so that you can do a few more. When you reach failure again, stretch your arm down toward your legs so that you can continue the exercise. By using this descending set strategy, you will be able to induce a very profound muscle fatigue, and typically one set will be enough for each side, which will save you time.

Variations

- You can perform a side crunch using an ab roller, which will help you find the correct range of motion and path for the movement.
- For a greater challenge, you can perform a side crunch on a roman chair machine.

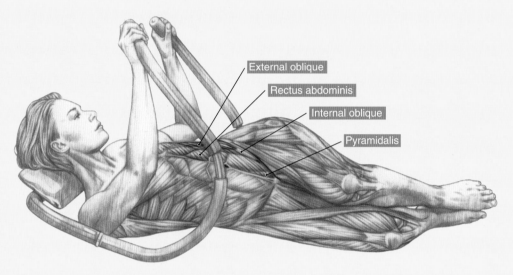

External oblique

Rectus abdominis

Internal oblique

Pyramidalis

▌ **Ab devices help you find the right contracting path**

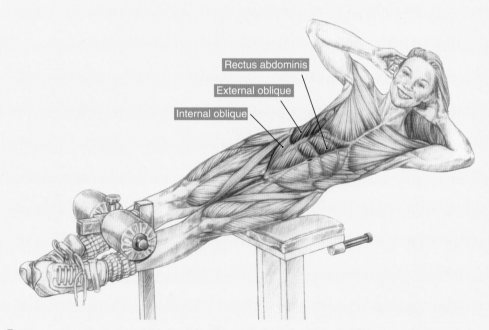

Rectus abdominis

External oblique

Internal oblique

▌ **Using a roman chair rather than the floor renders the exercise far more challenging**

- We strongly advise that you avoid standing side bend exercises that use dumbbells or a low cable pulley to train the obliques because they put unnecessary tension on the spine while placing the back in a very awkward position. These exercises are useful only in strength sports in which the spine needs to resist enormous tension. In that case, use a high pulley instead of a low one to avoid pressuring your lower back. Most important, do this movement only unilaterally; avoid using two dumbbells at the same time.

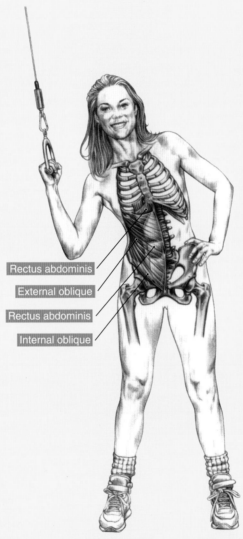

Rectus abdominis

External oblique

Rectus abdominis

Internal oblique

Side crunch variation with a high pulley, for strength sports

Twisting rotations belong in the isolated, single-joint exercise category. They do not recruit much of the muscle groups surrounding the obliques. Their main advantage is that they attack "love handles" better than any other exercise does.

How to Do It

- **Twist with a broomstick:** Sit on a bench or stand up while holding a broomstick on your shoulders. Slowly rotate from left to right using a reduced range of motion. Avoid jerky movements. We recommend that you choose a twist version that involves lateral resistance rather than resistance across your shoulders.

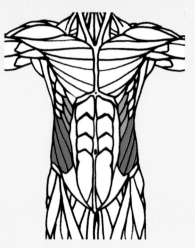

▌Main areas (in red) and secondary areas (in orange) targeted by the twist

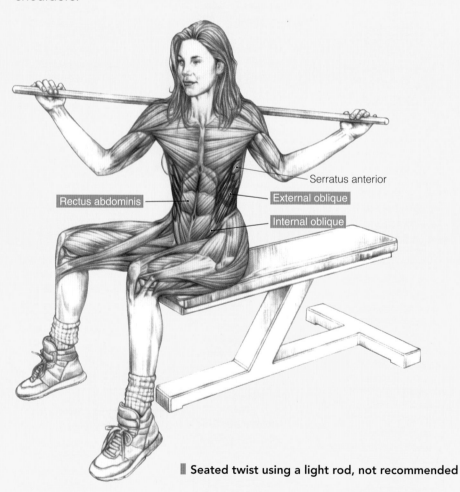

Serratus anterior

Rectus abdominis

External oblique

Internal oblique

▌Seated twist using a light rod, not recommended

- **Twist with an elastic band:** Attach a band to a fixed point that is at about shoulder height. Standing, grasp the band in both hands and step forward. The farther you step from where the band is attached, the greater the resistance will be.

  Standing with your legs apart to increase stability, rotate from right to left. Do not turn your torso more than 45 degrees. When you have finished working the right side, move immediately to the left side.

- **Twist with a machine:** Sit, stand, or kneel, depending on the equipment. Slowly rotate from left to right. Do not exaggerate the range of motion.

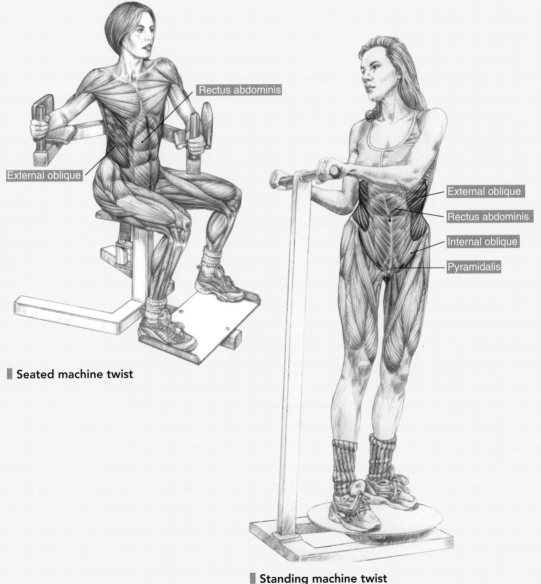

Rectus abdominis

External oblique

External oblique

Rectus abdominis

Internal oblique

Pyramidalis

▌ **Seated machine twist**

▌ **Standing machine twist**

Pro

- This is one of only a very few exercises that target love handles. Even so, love handles are not easy to get rid of. A proper diet and specific exercises will help.

Con

- This exercise can exacerbate back problems. If you have any back problems at all, do not perform the twist.

 Explosive movements with maximum range of motion can rapidly damage your spine.

Tips

- We recommend this exercise only with lateral resistance. Twisting wildly from side to side with a bar on the shoulders serves only to wear down the spine, especially when the bar is weighted.
- Don't try to rotate over the greatest range of motion possible. Use a reduced range of motion (no more than 10 in., or 25 cm, of rotation on each side). Slow your pace to make up for the short range of motion.
- Do this exercise slowly using long sets (e.g., 25 repetitions). Performing two to four sets every day will combat love handles.

FREE WEIGHTS OR MACHINE?

Machines provide a much better way to perform twists than a broomstick because they offer lateral resistance. Your obliques have to contract powerfully to oppose that resistance. Without a machine there is practically no resistance even if you perform hundreds of reps. If no machine is available, a simple elastic band can provide proper resistance.

Variations

- Do the twist while lying on the floor. Instead of moving your upper body, your legs perform the rotations. You can do the twist either with bent legs (easier) or straight legs (far more difficult).
- Twist while hanging on a pull-up bar with either bent legs (easier) or straight legs (much harder). This version provides the added advantage of decompressing the spine at the end of a workout.

Start position

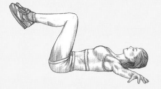

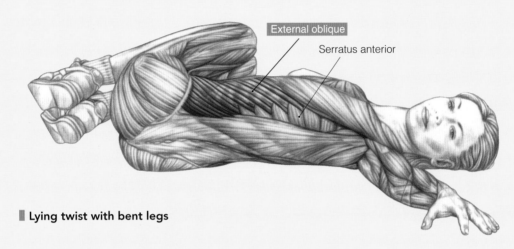

External oblique

Serratus anterior

Lying twist with bent legs

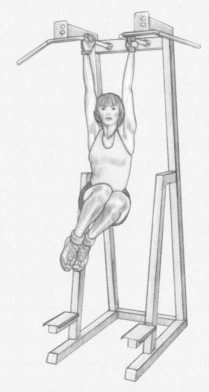

Hanging twist with bent legs

This static exercise targets the transversus abdominis and the obliques as well as many deep core muscles that support the spine.

How to Do It

Press your lower back as powerfully as possible against a wall with your feet about two feet (55 cm) away from the wall. Once in position, slowly bring your feet closer to the wall by taking very small steps. As you move, your lower back should remain in contact with the wall. When you reach the point where you are losing contact, stop moving your feet and hold the position for at least 20 seconds.

Pro

- Regular practice of this exercise helps to prevent back pain by training the core muscles that support the spine.

Con

- Because this exercise seems so easy, many women neglect it. This is a mistake.

Tip

- Although this exercise looks easy, you will feel a very strong contraction in your abdominal muscles. Because these core muscles are not used to such a powerful contraction, you will be amazed at how fast they get tired.

Variations

- If you cannot last 15 seconds in the standing position, do the exercise lying on the floor on your back with your legs bent at 90 degrees. Gently stretch your legs without arching your back. The objective here is to push the lumbar spine as strongly as possible against the floor. When you feel the lower back lift off the floor, stop extending your legs. Avoid pushing on your heels to keep your lower back against the floor. When this floor exercise becomes too easy, stand up to do it leaning against a wall.
- If the wall version becomes too easy, perform it while standing without the wall for support.

FREE WEIGHTS OR MACHINE?

No machine allows you to directly contract the transversus abdominis. You can easily do this exercise at home, whenever you want and as frequently as you want, because no equipment is required.

The plank works most of the core muscles, and there is no machine for this exercise. Thus, you can do it at home whenever you want and as frequently as you want.

How to Do It

Lie on the floor, facedown, resting on both your elbows and forearms and on the balls of your feet and your toes. Hold this static position for at least 15 seconds while keeping your body as straight as possible.

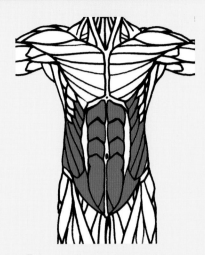

▌ **Red indicates the muscles worked during the plank**

Pros

- Because this isometric exercise requires no equipment, it can be done in very little time.

- This exercise is conducive to creating a friendly competition of seeing who among your friends can hold the plank the longest.

Con

- Isometric exercises are not the best for improving the aesthetic appearance of your abs. However, this exercise may be very appropriate for you if you require a strong core to compete in a combat or team contact sport.

❗ **Although holding your breath facilitates this exercise, you should refrain from stopping your breathing! If you find that breathing is challenging, exhale with tiny breaths.**

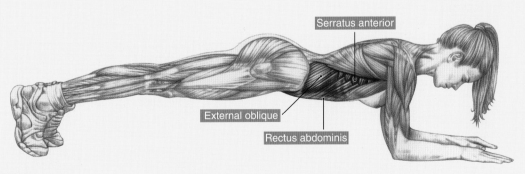

Serratus anterior

External oblique

Rectus abdominis

▌ **Elbow plank**

Tips

- If you experience any pain while putting your palms on the floor, make fists and put your hands in a neutral position (with only the pinkies in contact with the floor).

- If the weight of your head becomes too uncomfortable, bend your neck forward to let it rest against your hands.

- A gym mat (or at least a towel) will help you avoid pain in your forearms.

- Don't arch your lower back to make the exercise easier. If you bow your back excessively, you may pinch the intervertebral discs.

- A recent study suggests that the plank is three times more effective if you hollow your abdominal muscles (i.e., contract your glutes while tilting your pelvis slightly up and tucking your chest toward your abs).[3]

Variations

- To increase the difficulty of the exercise, you can have a partner place a weight plate on your back, or sit on you.

- To work the obliques, you can perform the exercise in a lateral position. If this version is too difficult, use your free hand for support by placing it on the floor in front of you.

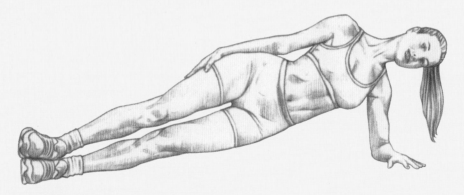

Side plank variation

To maintain a flat abdomen, do not stretch your abdominal muscles too much. On the other hand, if you are looking for a somewhat round belly, you can stretch them a little. Do not overdo the following stretch with too many repetitions or too great a range of motion.

Lie on the floor, facedown, resting on your abdomen. Using your hands, push your upper torso up. Hold this static position for at least 15 seconds.

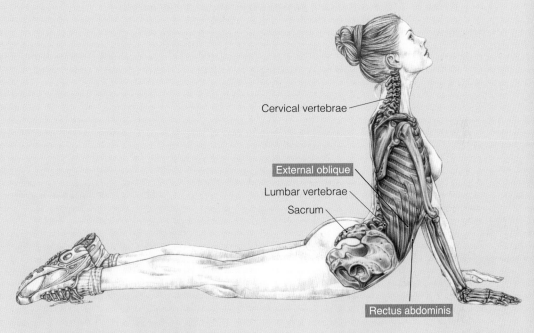

Cervical vertebrae

External oblique

Lumbar vertebrae

Sacrum

Rectus abdominis

▌ Prone ab stretch

Anatomy and Morphology

The deltoid is the muscle responsible for moving the arm in all directions. Aesthetically, your shoulders define your build. In a somewhat artificial manner, the deltoid is divided into three parts:

1. The front of the shoulder, which lifts the arm in front or overhead
2. The lateral part of the shoulder, which raises the arm to the side
3. The back of the shoulder, which pulls the arm backward

The deltoid is a single-joint muscle because it crosses only the shoulder joint. On the other hand, because of its various heads, you can work this muscle from plenty of angles by raising your arms in front of you, overhead, laterally, and posteriorly.

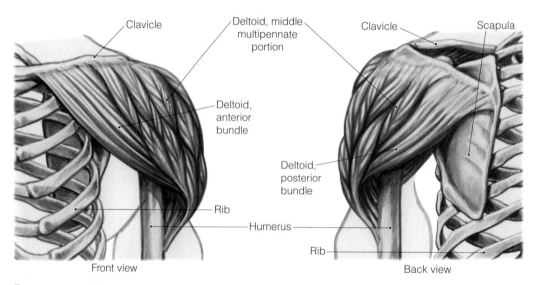

Front view

Back view

▌ Front view (left) and back view (right) of the deltoid muscles

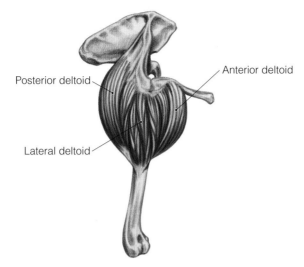

▌ Side view of the deltoid muscles

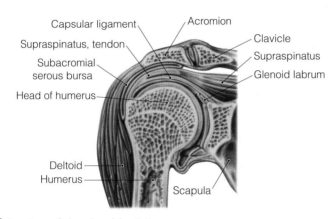

▌ Section of the shoulder joint

Take-Home Lesson for Women

Most sedentary females suffer from an anterior deltoid tilt. Such poor posture hides the breasts and often creates back pain. Weight training the shoulders will improve your posture, prevent back pain, and make you look even more attractive. Curved shoulders, created by pulling your arms backward, not only bring your breasts up but also make you appear taller.

Most women have a structural imbalance between the front and the back of the shoulders. This sitting-induced muscular disequilibrium can paradoxically be exacerbated by poorly designed weight training programs.

Scientists have measured this imbalance.[3] Compared to sedentary people, athletes with a good level of fitness have the following features:

- An average of 250 percent greater muscle mass on the front of the shoulder
- 150 percent greater muscle mass on the lateral part of the shoulder
- Only 10 to 15 percent greater muscle mass on the back of the shoulder

The most common shoulder exercises are the presses, which mostly stimulate the front delts. Because this anterior part of the deltoids is also strongly stimulated by chest exercises, the front shoulder is classically overstimulated and overdeveloped.

Furthermore, the front delt is also the area of the shoulder that responds best to weight training. The lateral and, especially, the rear delts are much more stubborn areas. They do gain strength, but toning them up is difficult. Moreover, it is even more difficult when you neglect them in favor of the anterior part of the deltoids.

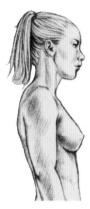
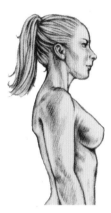

▌**Most sedentary females suffer from an anterior deltoid tilt (left). Weight training the shoulders will improve your posture (right) and prevent back pain.**

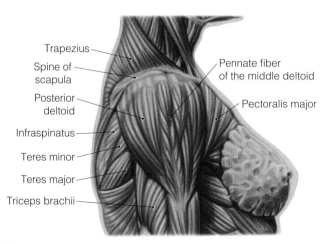

Trapezius

Spine of scapula

Posterior deltoid

Infraspinatus

Teres minor

Teres major

Triceps brachii

Pennate fiber of the middle deltoid

Pectoralis major

▌**Side view of the shoulder muscles**

Shoulder Exercises

There are three main categories of exercises for the shoulders from which women can benefit:

1. Lateral raise
2. Upright row
3. Bent-over lateral raise

Each category has several versions, which guarantees a great variety of movements and allows you to choose the ones that best suit both your anatomy and your goals.

The shoulder press is the fourth main category of shoulder exercises you will likely come across. But, for the following reasons, women should avoid the shoulder press:

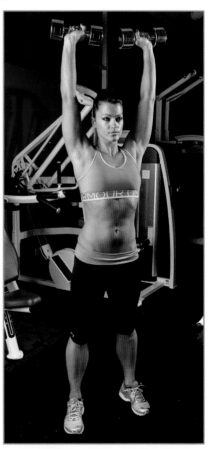

- The chest press already stimulates the front part of the shoulders. If you are seriously training your chest, it is not necessary to focus on the front of the shoulder, especially because this zone of the deltoid is the easiest to develop.
- Performing both chest and shoulder presses places unnecessary stress on the shoulder, elbow, and wrist joints, which is likely to translate into pain and injuries. Avoiding the shoulder press will save you time and lighten the burden on your joints.
- Overly developed front delts will deteriorate your posture.
- The typical weak area of the deltoids is the rear part. This is where you should focus your efforts.

▌ Dumbbell shoulder press. This isn't a bad exercise, and you will see many people performing it at the gym. However, it doesn't focus on the areas of the shoulder where women are typically weakest.

The goals of the warm-up sequence are to prepare the following muscles and joints for training and reduce the risk of injury:

- Shoulder joints
- Tendon of the long head of the biceps right in the middle of the front shoulder
- Lower back

Perform 20 to 30 easy repetitions of the following exercises using light weights. Move from one exercise to the next without any rest. If you do not feel that one cycle has warmed you up, feel free to perform a second cycle.

Once you have finished this overall warm-up cycle, move on to lateral raises using at least one light set to warm up your shoulders before handling heavier weights. If you are already warmed up because you have just finished training your back or your chest, there is no need to repeat this warm-up sequence, but you should still do at least two sets of a specific shoulder exercise as a warm-up.

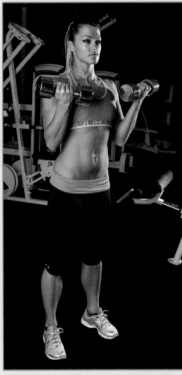

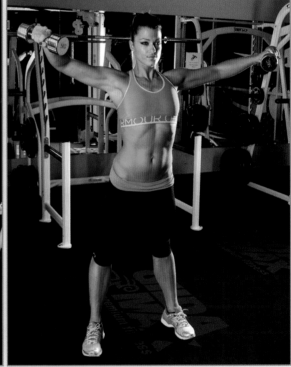

1. Biceps curl (see page 279)   2. Lateral raise (see page 196)

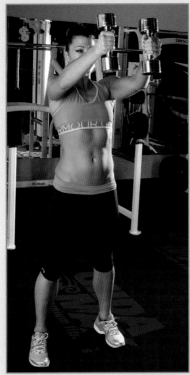

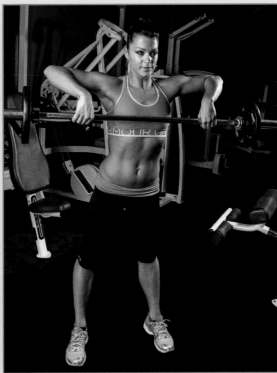

▌ 3. Front raise (see page 204)   ▌ 4. Upright row (see page 206)

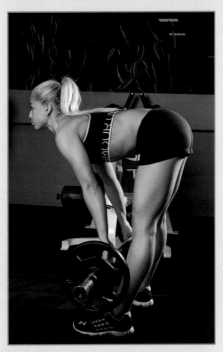

▌ 5. Stiff-leg deadlift (see page 114)

LATERAL RAISE

The lateral raise belongs in the isolating exercise category because only the shoulder joint is mobilized. As a consequence, the elevations do not recruit much muscle except the lateral part of the deltoids. This elevation of the arm is not very common in sports or in daily life, which explains why the role of the middle part of the shoulder is mostly aesthetic. The nice curve it provides justifies making the lateral raise the first exercise whenever shoulders are trained.

How to Do It

Grab two dumbbells or the handles of a cable or a machine. Raise your arms up while keeping them as straight as possible. At all times, keep them in line with your body. Raise your arms until they are parallel to the floor. Stop for one second, bring your arms down, and repeat the movement slowly.

The lateral raise can be performed with dumbbells, a machine, or a cable. Analyze the advantages and disadvantages of each version presented later in this section to choose the one that suits you best.

Pro

- Because the deltoids are very isolated muscles, they are conducive to drop sets when people want to work them deeply. You do not have to worry about any other muscle wearing out before the deltoids. As explained in part I, a descending set allows you to continue a set once you have reached fatigue without having to cheat. It involves briefly stopping the movement to rapidly remove around one third of the weight you are using and immediately resume your set. This allows you to continue the exercise and keep the muscle burn going. You can drop the load once or twice depending upon the level of muscular intensity you want to reach (the more drops you do per set, the more intense it is for your muscles).

Con

- Many people are tempted to cheat in this exercise so they can handle heavier weight, which is counterproductive.

- **Almost any kind of lateral raise puts pressure on the lower back. Therefore, it is a good idea to use a lifting belt to reduce this pressure as much as possible.**
- **If you cheat by oscillating your torso so that you can lift your arms, you will end up arching your lower back. This puts unnecessary pressure on your lower back.**

Tips

- With dumbbells or a cable, at all times during the exercise, the thumbs should be lower than the pinkie fingers so that you really focus your efforts on the lateral part of the deltoids.
- With dumbbells or a cable, bending the arms makes the exercise easier because your front shoulder comes into play; this is not desirable.
- You should be able to completely stop the movement with your arms parallel to the floor during the first few repetitions. If you cannot, you are using too much momentum to perform the movement and your weight is too heavy.
- With dumbbells, to train your shoulders really hard, start the exercise normally. At failure, move on immediately to dumbbell upright rows (discussed later). This is an advanced superset technique.

Pros of the Dumbbell Lateral Raise

- Equipment is readily available. You can use dumbbells or any kind of weight you can hold (e.g., water bottles).
- You can better target the middle shoulder–rear shoulder tie-in by changing the orientation of your upper body (i.e., bending a little bit forward or laterally). If you do so, keep your spine straight and use a lifting belt to protect your lower back.

Cons of the Dumbbell Lateral Raise

Even though this is the most popular version of the lateral raise (mostly because equipment is readily available), using dumbbells has more drawbacks than advantages. Following are three reasons the dumbbell lateral raise is not the best form of elevation:

- As you start raising your arms, most of the work is performed by the supraspinatus, not the deltoids. The deltoid muscles intervene only during the last two thirds of the movement. Because the supraspinatus is a fragile muscle, excessive stimulation is likely to result in chronic shoulder pain.

- The structure of resistance is very uneven with this exercise. The higher you lift your arms, the weaker your shoulder muscles become. The resistance the dumbbells provide becomes greater the higher you raise them. As a result, the difficulty of the exercise increases as the muscles are weakening. This poor match between the resistance pattern of the movement and the strength curve of the muscles makes this a less-than-optimal way to train the deltoids.

- The deltoids receive only a weak prestretch. Because the resistance from dumbbells diminishes rapidly when the arms come back to the body, the deltoids are not stretched very much.

Of all the lateral raise versions, the dumbbell lateral raise is the least productive and the most traumatic.

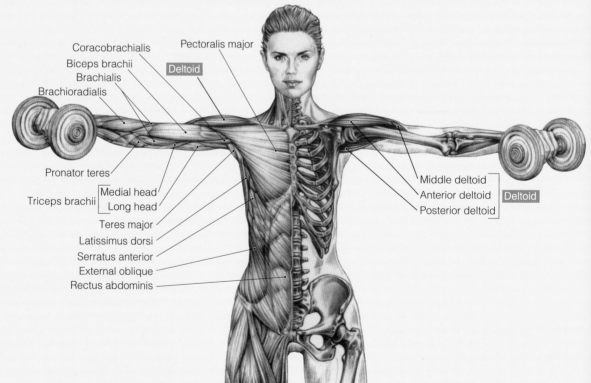

Coracobrachialis
Biceps brachii
Brachialis
Brachioradialis
Pectoralis major
Deltoid

Pronator teres
Triceps brachii — Medial head / Long head
Teres major
Latissimus dorsi
Serratus anterior
External oblique
Rectus abdominis

Middle deltoid
Anterior deltoid
Posterior deltoid
Deltoid

Start position

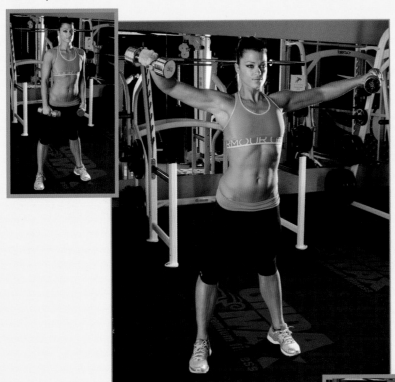

Dumbbell lateral raise

Dumbbell lateral raise with a lateral lean

Pro of the Machine Lateral Raise

- A good lateral raise machine is very effective because the resistance comes from the side. This is exactly the direction required to recruit the middle part of the deltoid. It is because the resistance of the dumbbells comes from the floor whereas free weights recruit the supraspinatus excessively.

Cons of the Machine Lateral Raise

- As with dumbbells, muscle prestretch is close to nonexistent with a machine, which reduces the range of motion of the exercise.
- On many lateral raise machines the spacing between the two moving arm axes cannot be adjusted. This spacing should correspond more or less to the width of your clavicles. Therefore, a single machine would not work for everyone. To get the maximum benefit from a machine that is either too wide or too narrow for you, do your set by raising only one arm at a time. This way, you can place your working shoulder exactly within the axis of rotation of the machine.
- Changing the orientation of the upper body to better target the middle shoulder–rear shoulder tie-in is often impossible.

Start position

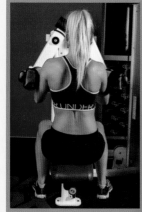

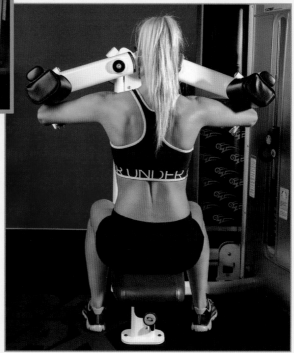

Machine lateral raise

Pros of the Cable Lateral Raise

- Low cable pulleys are more widely available than machines. They present a superior way of performing lateral raises in the safest manner possible.

- The direction of resistance corresponds more closely to the deltoid's work than with dumbbells. Ideally, you can adjust the height of the pulley by raising it a little below your knee so that the resistance comes exactly from the shoulder's pulling axis, not from the floor.

- The range of motion is increased because the pulley allows your arms to cross your torso in the bottom part of the movement. Your right arm can go much farther to the left and your left arm can go much farther to the right than either can with dumbbells or a machine.

- To better target the middle shoulder–rear shoulder tie-in, you can change the orientation of your upper body by bending a little bit forward or laterally. If you do so, keep your spine straight and use a lifting belt to protect your lower back.

Cons of the Cable Lateral Raise

- A cable makes it impractical to train both arms at the same time. You will have to work one arm at a time, which is time-consuming.

- When the pulley has to remain close to the floor, the resistance does not come from the side very much, which reduces the involvement of the deltoid in favor of the supraspinatus, which isn't a big improvement over dumbbells.

Start position

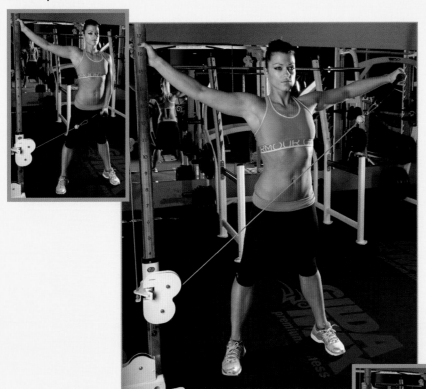

Cable lateral raise

Cable lateral raise with a lateral lean

Variations

- You can increase the range of motion of this exercise by raising your hands as high as possible rather than stopping them at shoulder level. If you do so, you should slowly rotate your hands so that your palms end up facing each other when the weights touch at the top of the movement. As you bring the weights down, slowly rotate the hands back so that your thumbs face the front as the dumbbells touch your legs. This variation will target your front shoulders and your upper trapezius more than the regular version.

- Work bilaterally if you are using dumbbells or a machine. Consider working unilaterally only if doing the exercise bilaterally makes you feel as though you're working the trapezius more than the deltoid muscles. This can happen for women with large clavicles.

- With dumbbells, you can do this exercise while sitting or standing. In general, your execution form is better when sitting than when standing. One approach is to begin this exercise sitting down and, at failure, stand up so that you can perform a few more repetitions.

- Instead of raising your arms to the side, lift them to the front using either dumbbells or a cable. This variation focuses on the front deltoids, which, as we explained earlier, makes this variation unnecessary for most women except to warm up the joints and the tendons. You can use either a neutral, hammer-style grip or a pronated grip with the palms down.

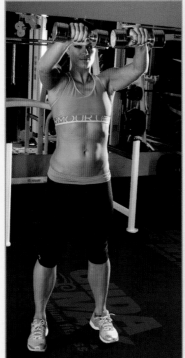 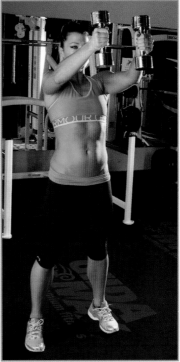

▌ Dumbbell front raise with a pronated grip

▌ Dumbbell front raise with a neutral hammer grip

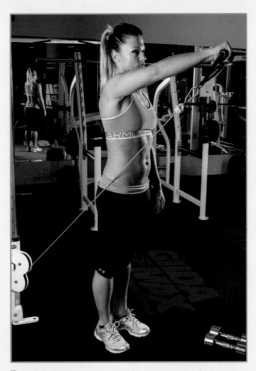

▌ Cable front raise with a pronated grip

The upright row belongs in the multiple-joint exercise category because the shoulder, elbow, and wrist joints are mobilized. As a result, the upright row recruits many muscles in addition to the shoulders: the upper trapezius, biceps, and forearms.

How to Do It

Stand holding a barbell, dumbbells, or pulley handle using a pronated, palms-down grip. Lift your arms while bending them, keeping your hands as close to your body as possible. You can lift the weight all the way to your chin, but many people prefer to lift the weight only as high as the chest.

Pro

- This is the only multiple-joint exercise for the shoulders that does not overstimulate the front shoulders.[1]

Con

- Not everyone can perform the upright row without incurring injuries. Some women's shoulders or wrist joints, or both, do not tolerate the rotations this exercise creates. If this is the case for you, replace the upright row with the lateral raise.

Do not raise your arms too high. Reduce the range of motion and stop the movement before your upper arms break parallel with the floor for these reasons:

- **The higher you raise your arms, the more the upper trapezius is recruited and the less the lateral delts are involved.**
- **Raising your arms too high forces your shoulder joints to rotate in an unhealthy manner. Your shoulders will start to rotate a little as your hands reach the level of your lower chest. Past that point, your shoulders are forced to rotate more and more. Extreme rotation will be required for your upper arms to break parallel with the floor.[2]**
- **As you raise your arms higher, your wrists have to withstand greater and greater stress to continue to hold on to the barbell.**

Pro of the Barbell Upright Row

- Balancing the weight is easier than with dumbbells.

Con of the Barbell Upright Row

- For many people, a straight bar causes an unnatural twisting of the wrist that can traumatize this joint. The higher you pull the barbell, the more you have to twist your wrists. An EZ bar (a.k.a. curl bar) can minimize this problem.

Start position

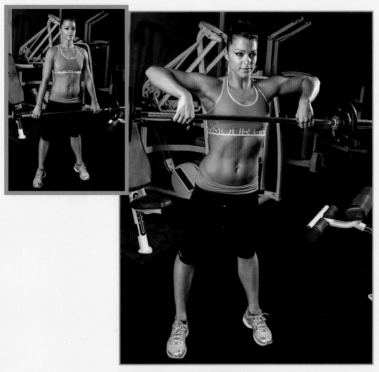

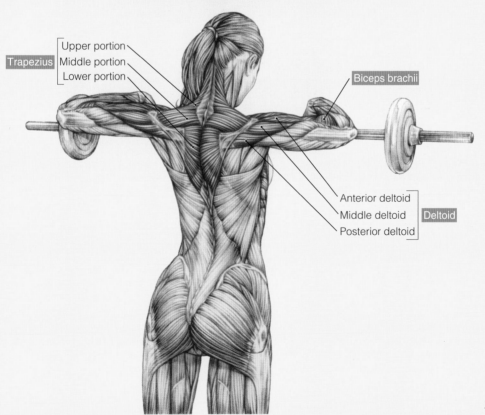

Upright row using a barbell

Trapezius
- Upper portion
- Middle portion
- Lower portion

Biceps brachii

Anterior deltoid
Middle deltoid
Posterior deltoid

Deltoid

Pro of the Smith Machine Upright Row

- Because the weight does not have to be balanced, this version is very beginner friendly.

Con of the Smith Machine Upright Row

- The hands are even less free to move than with a barbell, which increases the risk of twisting the wrists during the lift.

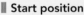
Start position

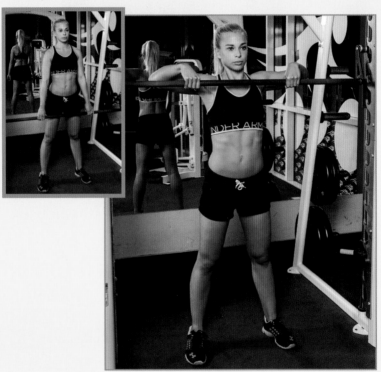

Machine upright row

FREE WEIGHTS OR MACHINE?

Because upright row machines are few and far between, we will not discuss them. Classically, the upright row can be performed using a barbell, dumbbells, a Smith machine, or a cable pulley. The muscular effects are very similar among these versions; only the impact on the joints differs.

Pro of the Dumbbell Upright Row

- The hand is completely free to move, which minimizes any unnatural twisting of the wrists and allows you to rotate your hands to optimize the recruitment of the lateral part of the deltoids.

Con of the Dumbbell Upright Row

- Because of the freedom of movement of both arms, balancing the weight is challenging, which may be difficult for beginners. However, getting used to controlling the dumbbells so that both arms are lifted simultaneously happens quickly.

Pros of the Cable Upright Row

- A low cable is much gentler for the shoulder joint than free weights are.
- Performing this exercise while lying on the floor greatly minimizes the pressure placed on the spine. If you suffer from mild back pain and insist on training your shoulders, this is the version of choice. In any case, do not arch your low back. Keep it in contact with the floor at all times.

Con of the Cable Upright Row

- If you are using a straight bar, you face the same wrist problems that you would with a barbell. If possible, use an EZ bar instead.

Tips

- If you feel your trapezius muscle too much, you may want to try the unilateral version, either with a dumbbell or a cable. Other than that, even if it is easy to perform this exercise one arm at a time, working both arms at once saves time.
- You must place your hands at the proper width to recruit the deltoids rather than the trapezius. Following are general rules:
  - The wider the grip is, the less the trapezius will be involved.
  - The higher you pull the bar, dumbbells, or pulley handle, the more your trapezius will come into play.
- Arching your lower back permits you to handle heavier weight, but it also makes you more prone to spinal injuries.

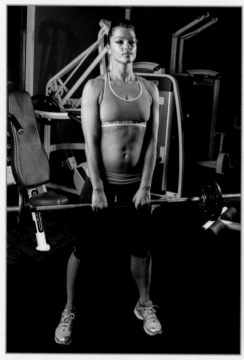

▍A narrow grip involves the trapezius more

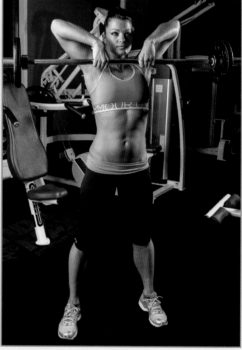

▍A higher pull involves the trapezius more

The bent-over lateral raise belongs in the isolating exercise category because only the shoulder joint is mobilized. Yet, this exercise recruits many of the muscle groups surrounding the deltoids—namely, the upper back (trapezius, rhomboids, and part of the latissimus dorsi) as well as the long head of the triceps.

Bent-over laterals can be performed with dumbbells, a cable, or a machine. Analyze the advantages and disadvantages of each version later in this section to choose the one that suits you best.

How to Do It: Dumbbells and Cable

With dumbbells or a cable, lean forward so that your torso forms a 90-degree to 120-degree angle to the floor. Grab the dumbbells or cable handle using a pronated, palms-down grip (thumbs toward each other). A neutral grip (hammer grip with thumbs facing the front) can also be adopted with the cable handle. Lift your arms to the sides as high as possible while keeping them as straight as possible. Hold the contracted position for one to two seconds; then lower the weights.

How to Do It: Rear Deltoid Machine

Sit in the machine and make sure the pad does not compress your breasts excessively, which may become painful as the set goes on. Depending on the machine, you can adopt either a neutral (hammer) or pronated (palms-down) grip. Pull your arms to the rear as far as possible. Hold the contracted position for one to two seconds before bringing your arms back to the front.

Pro

- The rear deltoid is the most neglected and most underdeveloped part of the shoulder. As discussed in the introduction of this section, women often neglect the backs of their shoulders. It is wise to work the rear of the shoulders as often as possible with the bent-over lateral raise. This is a key exercise for this area.

Con

- The bent-over position is not comfortable. Be sure that your stomach is not too full of food or water when you start this exercise.

With dumbbells, your lower back is put at risk. If you have access to a machine, you will get the same results as with dumbbells, if not better, while training much more safely.

Pro of the Dumbbell Bent-Over Lateral Raise

- Equipment is readily available. You can use dumbbells or any kind of weight you can hold (e.g., water bottles).

Cons of the Dumbbell Bent-Over Lateral Raise

- This version places significant tension on the lower back.
- The bent-over position may not be comfortable.
- The range of motion of the exercise is limited by a lack of resistance in the stretched part of the movement.

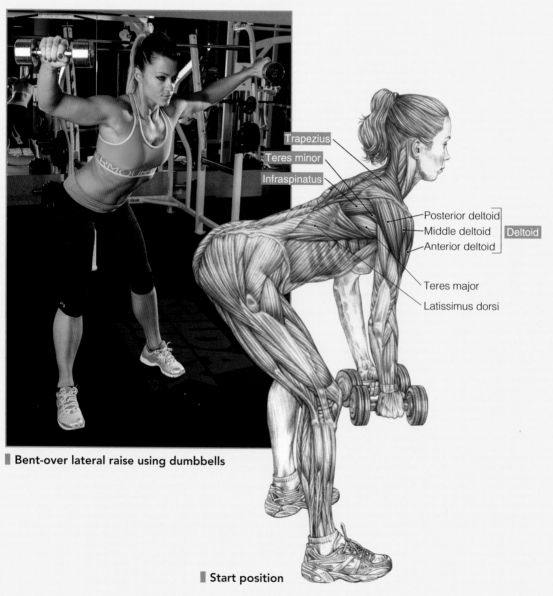

Bent-over lateral raise using dumbbells

Start position

Pro of the Cable Bent-Over Lateral Raise

- Because of the pronounced stretch at the bottom of the movement, a cable allows a much longer range of motion than dumbbells and even machines. Because the upper back region is difficult to develop, using the greatest range of motion possible, especially by increasing the stretched portion of the movement, is very effective.

Cons of the Cable Bent-Over Lateral Raise

- The cable makes it very impractical to train both arms at the same time. You will need to work one arm at a time, which will increase the duration of your training.
- Unnecessary tension is placed on the lower back.
- The bent-over position may not be comfortable.

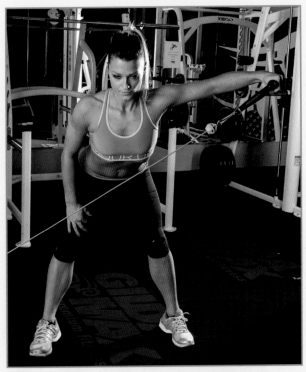

Bent-over lateral raise using a low pulley

Pros of the Rear Deltoid Machine Lateral Raise

- Machines are much safer for the lower back because most of them have you perform the movement in a seated position. As a result, the pressure on the spine is reduced compared to a bent-over standing position.
- The seated position is also much more comfortable because breathing is easier than when you bend over to lift weights.
- Some machines have you lie down but provide a back support to take the pressure off the lower back. However, they may not be very comfortable because your rib cage is blocked by a pad or a bench.

Con of the Rear Deltoid Machine Lateral Raise

- Machines are not readily available. If you do not have access to one, use a low pulley and work one arm at a time. Only in the absence of either a machine or a pulley do we recommend the dumbbell bent-over lateral raise.

▌ Start position

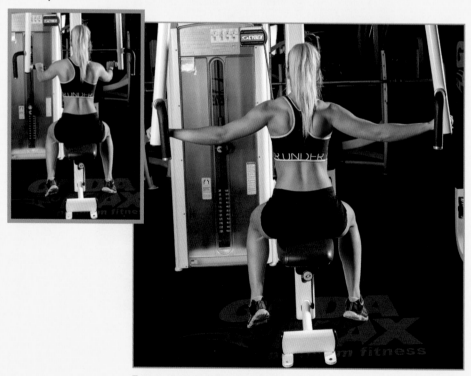

▌ Rear deltoid machine lateral raise

Tips

- Perform this exercise using descending sets to make sure you really work the muscle to the maximum.

- Keep your head very straight and look straight ahead with your gaze slightly upward to keep your back perfectly aligned.

- The movement is easier if you do not keep your arms perfectly perpendicular to your torso. Drifting them downward allows you to use heavier weights, but it does not isolate your rear shoulders nearly as well. So, make sure you raise your arms straight up to your sides even if you have to lighten your weight to do so.

STRETCH THE SHOULDERS

It is very important to stretch the shoulders, especially the front parts, which tend to lack flexibility. The rear parts can be stretched also, but doing so is less important. Because of the anterior deltoid tilt that most sedentary females suffer from, the rear part of the shoulders is constantly overstretched while the front part is perpetually shortened. Stretching is a powerful tool to improve your posture, especially by targeting the front part of the delts. It is nearly impossible to stretch the lateral part of the deltoids because your body interferes with the arm movement.

- To stretch the front of the shoulder, stand with one hand grabbing the wrist of the other arm behind your back. Then, pull your arm as far as possible behind you with your hand. Hold the stretched position for 10 to 30 seconds and then repeat with the other arm.

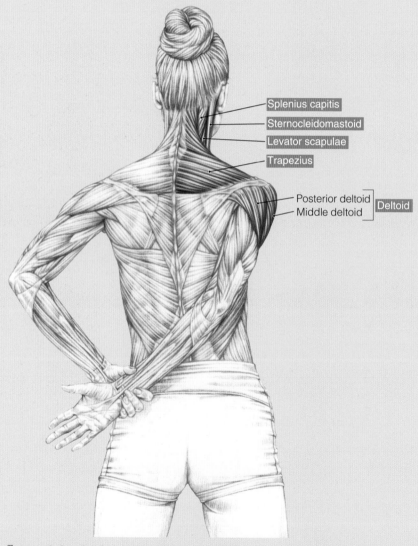

Splenius capitis
Sternocleidomastoid
Levator scapulae
Trapezius
Posterior deltoid
Middle deltoid
Deltoid

▌ Stretch for the front part of the shoulder

- To stretch the rear part of the shoulder, stand with your left arm straight in front of you. Grab the left elbow with the right hand. Pull your left arm toward your chest as much as you can. Hold the position for 10 to 30 seconds and then repeat with the other arm.

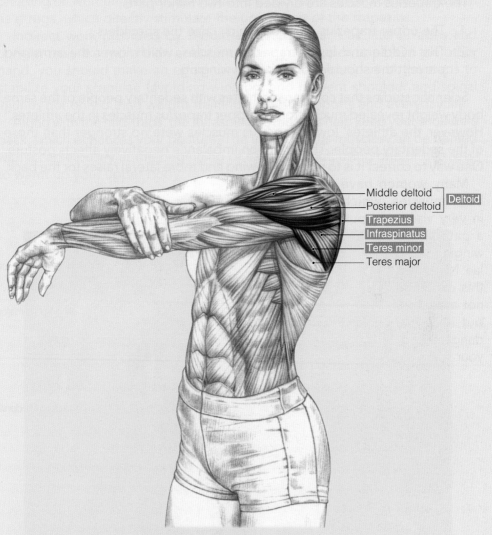

Middle deltoid
Posterior deltoid — Deltoid
Trapezius
Infraspinatus
Teres minor
Teres major

▌ Stretch for the rear part of the shoulder

The goals of the warm-up sequence are to prepare the following for training and reduce the risk of injury:

- All upper-body joints
- Tendon of the long head of the biceps and the biceps muscle
- Triceps
- Lower back

Perform 20 to 30 easy repetitions of the following exercises with light weights. Move from one exercise to the next without any rest. If you do not feel that one cycle has warmed you up, feel free to perform a second cycle.

Once you have finished this overall warm-up cycle, move on to your first back exercise using at least two light sets to specifically warm up your back before handling heavier weights. If you are already warmed up because you have just finished training your chest or your shoulders, there is no need to repeat this warm-up sequence, but you should still do the two light sets of a specific back exercise as a warm-up.

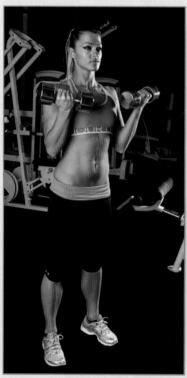 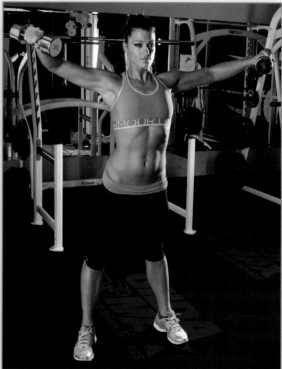

1. Biceps curl (see page 276)   **2. Lateral raise (see page 196)**

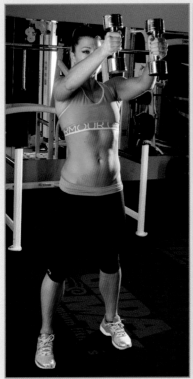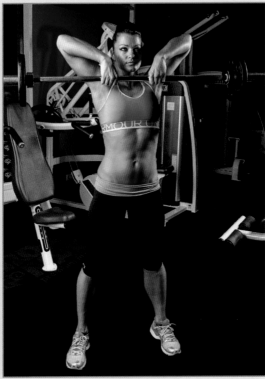

3. Front raise (see page 205)   4. Upright row (see page 206)

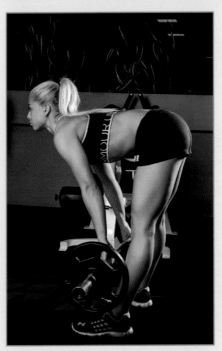

5. Stiff-leg deadlift (see page 114)

Upper Back Exercises

There are three main categories of exercises for the upper back from which women can benefit:

1. Row
2. Pull-down
3. Pullover

Each category has several versions, which guarantees a great variety of movements and allows you to choose the ones that best suit both your anatomy and your goals.

The row belongs in the basic, multiple-joint exercise category because both the shoulder and the elbow joints are mobilized. As a result, rowing recruits many muscles in addition to the entire back: the rear shoulders, the biceps, the long head of the triceps, and the forearms. The row is considered a good starting exercise because it stimulates many muscle groups of the upper body.

How to Do It

- **Dumbbell row:** Lean forward so that your torso forms a 90- to 120-degree angle to the floor. Hold two dumbbells in a neutral grip with the thumbs forward. Some people prefer to have their thumbs slightly turned in, and others like them slightly turned out. Choose whichever position allows you the most powerful muscle contraction.

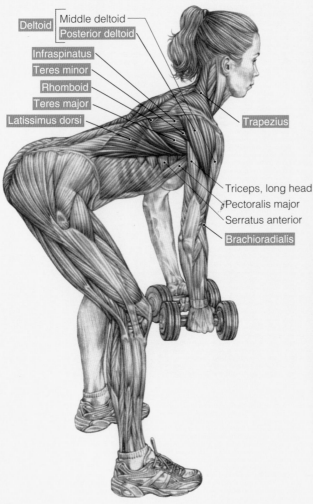

Deltoid — Middle deltoid
— Posterior deltoid
Infraspinatus
Teres minor
Rhomboid
Teres major
Latissimus dorsi

Trapezius

Triceps, long head
Pectoralis major
Serratus anterior
Brachioradialis

▌Start position

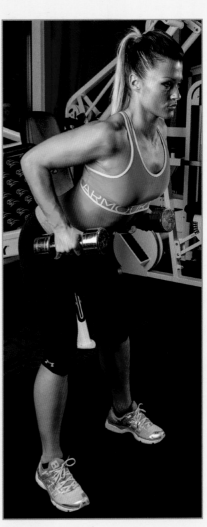

▌Dumbbell row

223

- **Barbell row:** Lean forward so that your torso forms a 90- to 120-degree angle to the floor. Grab a barbell with a supinated or pronated grip (see the Variations section for information to make the best choice for you).

▌ **Start position**

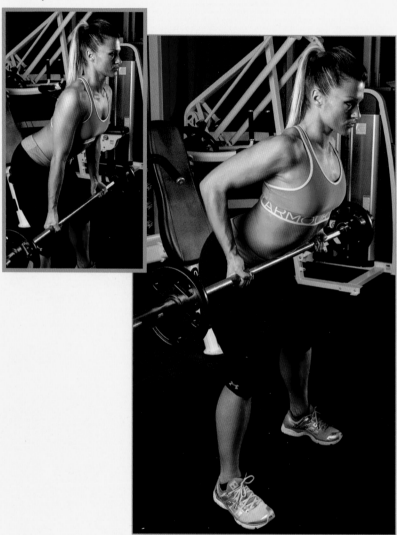

▌ **Barbell row, supinated grip**

- **Cable machine row:** Adjust the seat of the machine, and grab the movement arms or handles using a neutral, supinated, or pronated grip.

Start position, neutral grip

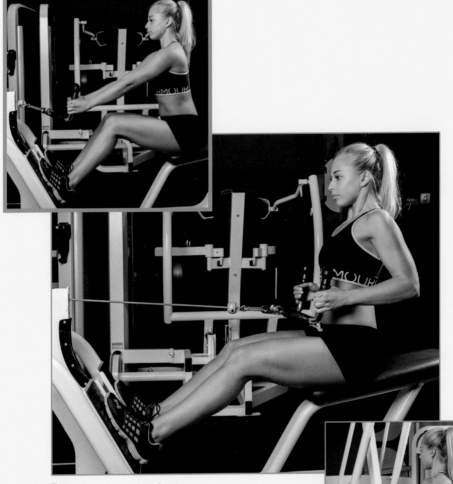

Cable row, neutral grip

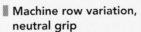

Machine row variation, neutral grip

ROW

For all versions of the row, pull your arms along your body, bending them and bringing your elbows as far back as possible. Squeeze your shoulder blades together and maintain the contracted position for one to two seconds; then lower the weights and repeat.

As a general rule, you should pull your hands back to your navel. Some people pull to their chests, and others, a little lower, near their thighs.

Pros

- Rowing works the muscles of the entire back, particularly the middle and lower trapezius.
- Rowing is better than pull-downs at targeting the muscles that enhance posture.
- Rowing is better than pull-downs at protecting the lower back.

Cons

- Leaning forward can interfere with breathing when working intensely.
- The leaning position places the spine in a precarious position.

- **Rowing with both hands, especially with heavy weights, can put the back at risk. You can reduce this risk by not bending to the often-recommended 90 degrees. Instead, lift your torso only until it is at a 120-degree angle to the floor. Because you may find it easier to feel your upper back muscles work from this position, you may feel stronger using it.**
- **The row is easier when you arch your back, but doing so is far riskier for your spine.**

Tips

- Keep a continuous tension in your back muscles so you do not straighten your arms too much in the stretched position. Doing so will prevent the biceps and shoulder injuries that can occur from repeatedly straightening the arms too much.
- Keep your head straight, especially during the contraction phase of the exercise. Avoid turning your head to either side.

Variations

- Unilateral work is very popular with dumbbells and machine rowing because it greatly increases the range of motion. Unfortunately, it also lengthens your workout. However, if you do not feel your upper back contract well with bilateral rowing, it is wise to switch to unilateral rows considering the importance of strengthening the back muscles.

- With dumbbells and barbells, and on some machines, you can alter your grip. A neutral grip (thumbs facing up) provides the most strength and places your arms in a way that makes you less prone to damaging your biceps. If you do not like it, try a supinated grip (palms facing up). In that case, it is of the utmost importance not to lengthen your arms completely in the stretched portion of the movement, because doing so will place your biceps in a very vulnerable position. A pronated grip (palms facing down) is possible, but it provides the least amount of strength and thus is not recommended.

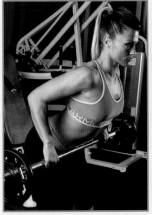 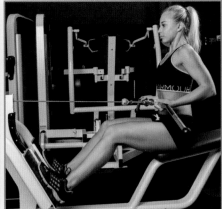

▌ Barbell row, pronated grip (not recommended)

▌ Cable row, supinated grip

FREE WEIGHTS OR MACHINE?

Some machines are pretty good at replicating the rowing movement. The main difference between free-weight rows and machine rows is that most machines attempt to protect the lower back from the excessive pressure the spine receives in the bent-over position. Of course, because machines guide the trajectory of the arms, they do not offer the variety of pathways dumbbells do. However, for beginners who might not have strong lower backs or who lack the ability to strongly recruit their lumbar muscles, machine rowing is a good way to begin back training.

PULL-DOWN

The pull-down belongs in the multiple-joint exercise category because both the shoulder and the elbow joints are mobilized. As a result, the pull-down recruits many muscles in addition to the back: the rear shoulders, the biceps, the long head of the triceps, and the forearms.

How to Do It

Sit at a high-pulley machine and grab the bar with supinated hands (palms up, pinkie fingers facing each other). Your hands should be about shoulder-width apart. You can also use a pronated grip (palms down, thumbs facing each other) to change the angle of attack for this exercise, as shown. In that case, use a wider grip. Vary the position of your hands until you find the one that works best for you.

Using a close grip with supinated hands is easier than using a wider grip in pronation; however, the biceps work more and the back works less with this version. If you are a beginner, a supinated, close grip is good to use until your strength increases.

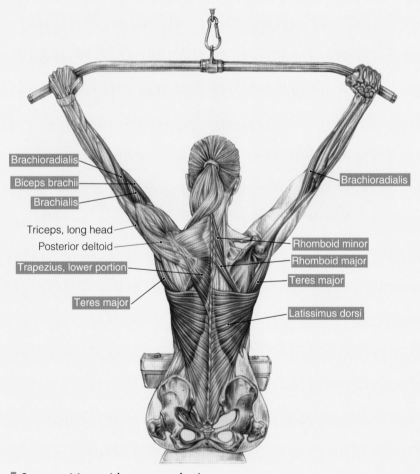

❚ Start position; wide, pronated grip

A neutral grip is also an option; this grip allows you to be stronger than in a pronated position. The back muscles stretch more in the bottom position, but the range of motion is more limited in the contracted position.

Pull the bar down at least to your forehead. If you feel comfortable enough, bring the bar to your upper chest. Maintain the contracted position for one second before slowly returning the bar to its starting position. Do not straighten your arms completely before repeating.

You have the option of bringing the bar in front of or behind the head. This latter version is the most difficult and the most traumatizing to the shoulder joints, and we don't recommend it.

▌ **Pull-down to the fore-head with a narrow, supinated grip**

▌ **Pull-down to the upper chest with a neutral grip and double row handle**

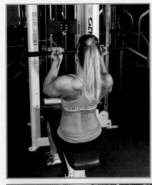
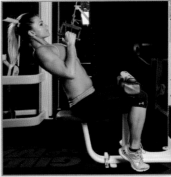

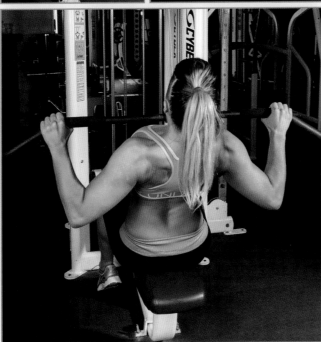

▌ **Pull-down to the upper chest**

PULL-DOWN

Never straighten your arms when performing the pull-down or the chin-up variation described later. Doing so creates an extreme stretch that puts the biceps and shoulders at risk of tearing. Instead, maintain continuous tension during the entire stretching part of the exercise. Some people straighten their arms to rest between repetitions. If you choose to do this, keep in mind that your shoulder ligaments are in a vulnerable position when you are hanging; take extra care to resume the pull-down or chin-up smoothly, without jerking.

Chin-Up Variation

As you gain strength from performing machine pull-downs, you will be ready to do chin-ups on a bar. To do so, grab the bar using a supinated grip (palms up) and with your hands about shoulder-width apart. Pull your feet up behind you to create a 90-degree angle between your calves and thighs. Cross your legs until your right foot pushes against your left ankle. Ensure a good grip on the bar by placing your thumb on your index finger (and your middle finger if your thumb is long enough).

Using your back muscles, pull yourself up until your forehead reaches the bar. If you can, bring your chin (or your neck) to the bar while tilting your head back. Hold the contracted position for one second before coming down slowly. Do not straighten your arms completely. Maintain continuous tension to prevent injuries.

With chin-ups, your body tends to sway. To avoid this problem and keep your body straight, squeeze your buttocks together hard and push your right foot against your left ankle. This extra rigidity will keep you from swaying.

To increase the challenge when you can easily do 12 to 15 chin-ups with your body weight, you can add resistance by squeezing a dumbbell or medicine ball between your calves or your thighs.

Pros

- In very little time, pull-downs work a very large section of the muscles in the torso.
- Pull-downs allow you to choose the resistance you want to apply to your muscles. You can increase this resistance by a small amount set after set, which is much harder to do with chin-ups.

Con

- Many women, unfortunately, are unable to pull themselves up using a horizontal bar, which can be frustrating. To cope with this situation, chin-up machines can be very handy because they allow you to choose the resistance that suits your strength level so you can do a normal set.

The pullover belongs in the isolated, single-joint exercise category because only the shoulder joint is mobilized. Even though it involves only a single joint, the pullover recruits major muscles such as the latissimus dorsi and the lower traps and, to a lesser extent, the pectoralis and the long head of the triceps. The serratus anterior muscle might also come into play. Despite this large recruitment, the pullover is more a stretching exercise than a muscle-building one. It is a good way to increase the flexibility of your rib cage.

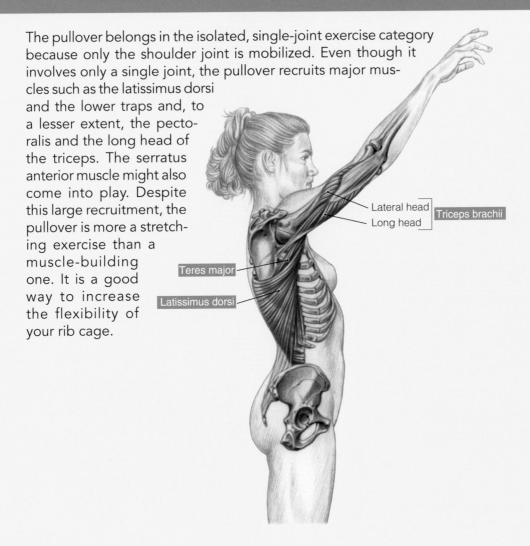

Lateral head
Long head
Triceps brachii

Teres major

Latissimus dorsi

FREE WEIGHTS OR MACHINE?

Machine and free-weight pullovers are very different. Machines provide less of a stretch than free weights do, but the stability they provide allows you to use heavier weights over a greater range of motion. As a result, machines provide more toning than free weights do.

With free weights, the emphasis should be on the stretching part as the resistance is only provided over half the range of motion. This is because the more you bring your arms over your body, the less resistance you place on the targeted muscles.

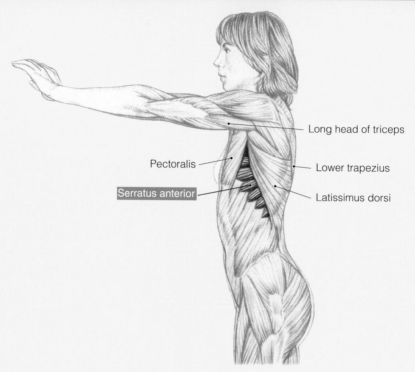

Long head of triceps

Pectoralis

Lower trapezius

Serratus anterior

Latissimus dorsi

How to Do It: Dumbbell

Lie supine on a bench with your head at the edge of the bench. Hold a dumbbell with both hands in a neutral grip (thumbs toward the floor) or a pronated grip (thumbs touching), bend your arms to 90 degrees, and move your arms above your head.

Keeping your arms bent, lower them behind your head. Bring them as low as possible and then raise them back up. Do not bring the weight all the way back up. Raise it only as long as you feel resistance; if this resistance disappears, you went too far to maintain continuous tension.

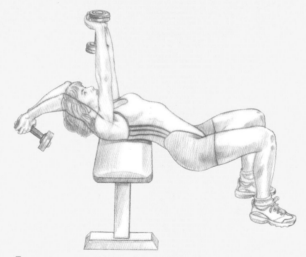

Dumbbell pullover on a bench

How to Do It: Machine

Adjust the seat and grab the movement arm or bar using a pronated, supinated, or neutral grip (this will depend on the type of machine you are using). Pull the arms along the length of your body with the strength of your lats so that your elbows get as close as possible to the rear of your obliques. Maintain the contracted position for one to two seconds while squeezing your shoulder blades together before raising your arms again and repeating the movement.

If you do not have access to a machine, you can use a high pulley. With your arms straight and your hands close to each other, bring the bar down, keeping your arms straight.

▌ Start position

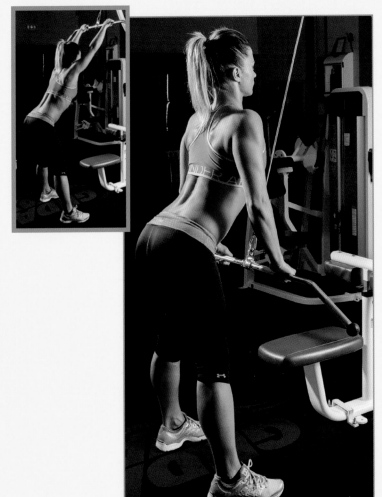

▌ Pullover using a high pulley

▌ Machine pullover

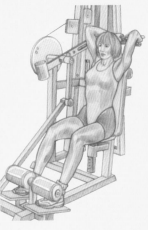

233

Pro

- If you feel only your biceps working and not your back muscles when performing chin-ups, pull-downs, or rows, then pullovers can really help you. This is because the biceps do not interfere during pullovers. Pre-exhausting your back muscles by starting with the pullover will allow you to feel your lats working more and your biceps less during pull-downs or rows.

Con

- Because pullovers place the shoulder joints in a relatively unstable position, you should avoid using too much weight. To increase the work, increase the number of repetitions rather than the weight.

❗ Do not stretch your shoulder to the point of discomfort at the joint level. Make sure you move the weight very slowly so that you can control the intensity of the stretch. Do not jerk the weight.

Tips

- Don't train your triceps before starting pullovers; if you do, you run the risk of them being too tired, which will prevent the lats from working as hard as they are supposed to. By either keeping your arms straight or bending them a little, you can modify your position to minimize the recruitment of your triceps.
- If you are using an adjustable dumbbell, make sure any weights are securely attached because you do not want them to fall off when they are above your head!
- With dumbbells, as your muscles tire toward the end of the set, you may tend to pull more with one arm than the other. Try to pull in as perfect a line as possible to avoid damaging your shoulder joints.

Variation

- Because the pullover works the latissimus dorsi muscles through stretching, you must try to go down as low as possible without forcing your shoulders. We do not recommend this extreme position on a machine, but with a light dumbbell, this is possible. In that case, to do so, instead of lying on the bench, you can lie across it so that both your shoulders and your hips can go down as you bring the dumbbell down (see the bench illustration earlier on page 232). This advanced version is only recommended after several weeks of regular pullover training.

Hold the following stretches for 10 to 20 seconds while breathing normally before moving to the other side of your body.

- Standing or seated, clasp your hands with your arms straight up. Bend over to one side pulling your arms up as much as possible. Hold the stretch for at least 15 seconds before bending toward the other side.

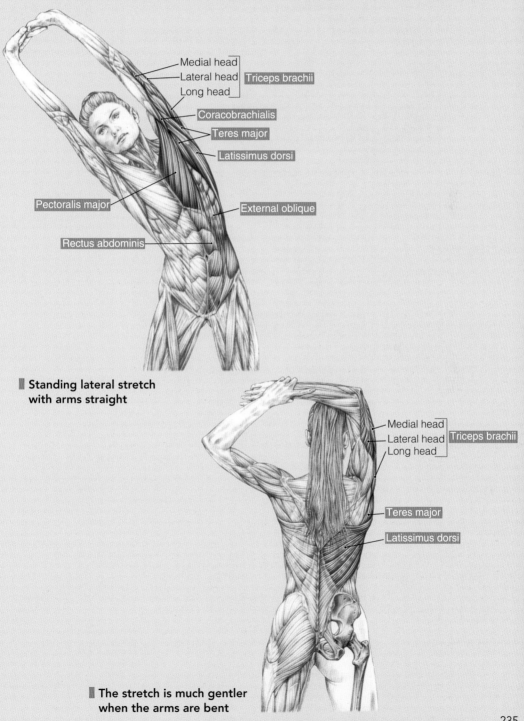

Medial head
Lateral head — Triceps brachii
Long head

Coracobrachialis

Teres major

Latissimus dorsi

Pectoralis major

External oblique

Rectus abdominis

**▌Standing lateral stretch
with arms straight**

Medial head
Lateral head — Triceps brachii
Long head

Teres major

Latissimus dorsi

**▌The stretch is much gentler
when the arms are bent**

- Gently stretching the neck is a good idea to relieve tension in the upper traps area.

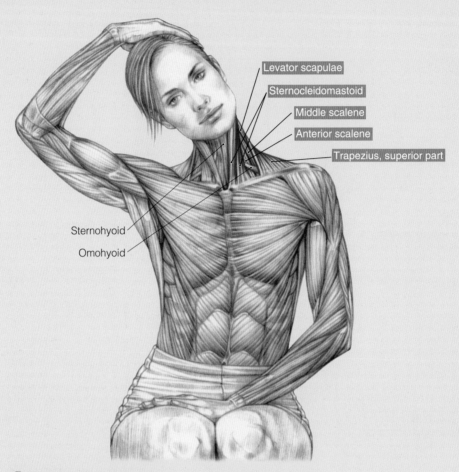

Levator scapulae

Sternocleidomastoid

Middle scalene

Anterior scalene

Trapezius, superior part

Sternohyoid

Omohyoid

▍**Seated neck stretch**

Anatomy and Morphology

The lumbar muscles support the spine. When they are sufficiently developed, these muscles can take pressure off the spine.

The lumbar muscles are also responsible for bringing the torso upright from a forward-leaning position. In this task, the lumbar muscles rarely work alone; they typically contract along with the glutes and the hamstrings.

Studies have shown that lower back pain is directly related to weak lumbar musculature.[1] Strengthening the lower back muscles is the best way to reduce lower back pain and prevent future back pain. So, it is much wiser to train your back as a preventive measure rather than once back pain has begun to affect your well-being.

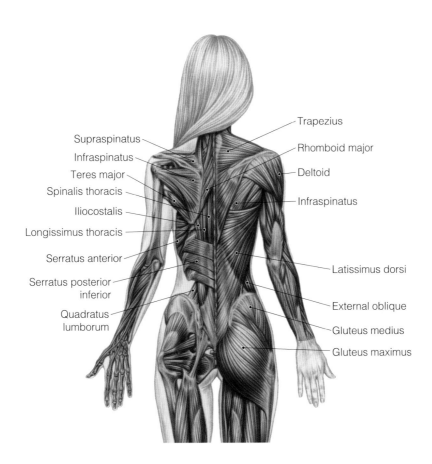

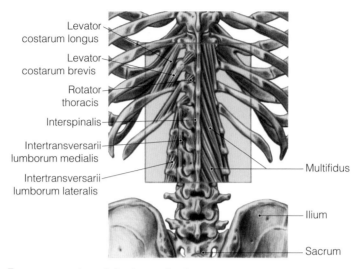

Levator costarum longus

Levator costarum brevis

Rotator thoracis

Interspinalis

Intertransversarii lumborum medialis

Intertransversarii lumborum lateralis

Multifidus

Ilium

Sacrum

▌ Deep muscles of the lower back

Take-Home Lesson for Women

The spine is a weak structure, especially as it ages. Weight training can both strengthen your muscles and increase your bone density, but it can also endanger your spine. Always be careful when you perform exercises that place pressure on your spinal column.

Warm Up the Lower Back

Starting your workout with lumbar exercises is generally not recommended. It is wiser to end your training with lumbar exercises to avoid tiring the muscles that support your spine before your workout. Therefore, when you start your lumbar exercises, you should already be fully warmed up.

Lower Back Exercises

There are two main categories of exercises for the lumbar muscles from which women can benefit:

1. Deadlift
2. Hyperextension

Each category has several versions, which guarantees a great variety of movements and allows you to choose the ones that best suit both your anatomy and your goals.

The deadlift belongs in the multiple-joint exercise category because the hip, the knee, and the ankle joints are mobilized. As a result, the deadlift recruits many muscles in addition to the lumbar muscles: the latissimus dorsi, the glutes, the hamstrings, and the quads.

The deadlift is considered a good overall exercise because it stimulates so many muscle groups throughout the body. If you do not have much time to train, the deadlift will strengthen several muscles in the limited amount of time you do have.

How to Do It: Dumbbells

With your feet shoulder-width apart and with a dumbbell beside each foot, bend your knees so your thighs are about perpendicular to the floor. Lift the dumbbells while keeping your back level. A semi-pronated grip, somewhere between a neutral grip (thumbs forward) and a pronated grip (thumbs facing each other) is ideal, but use whichever feels the most natural.

Allow your back to arch slightly backward to respect the natural curve of your spine. Push down through your heels and pull with your back to stand up. Synchronize the movements of your legs and back as much as possible. From the standing position, bend your legs while leaning to return to the start position.

▍**Start position**

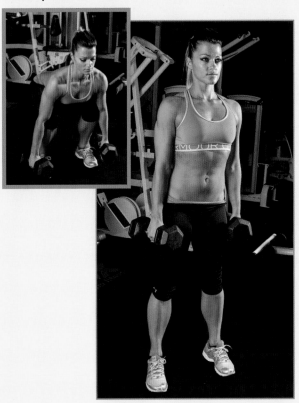

▍**Dumbbell deadlift**

How to Do It: Barbell

With your feet shoulder-width apart, bend your knees so your thighs are about perpendicular to the floor. Keeping your back level, use a pronated grip (thumbs facing each other) to grab the barbell from the floor. To handle heavier weights, place one hand in a supinated position with the palm up.

Allow your back to arch slightly backward to respect the natural curve of your spine. Push down through your heels and pull with your back to stand up. Synchronize the movements of your legs and back as much as possible. From the standing position, bend your legs while leaning forward to return to the start position.

‖ Start position

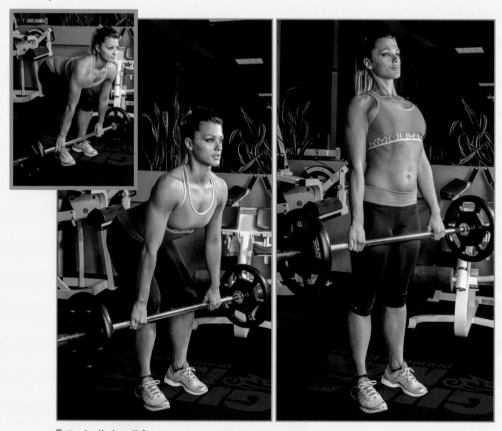

‖ Barbell deadlift

Mixed grip (left) and pronated grip (right)

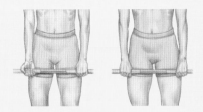

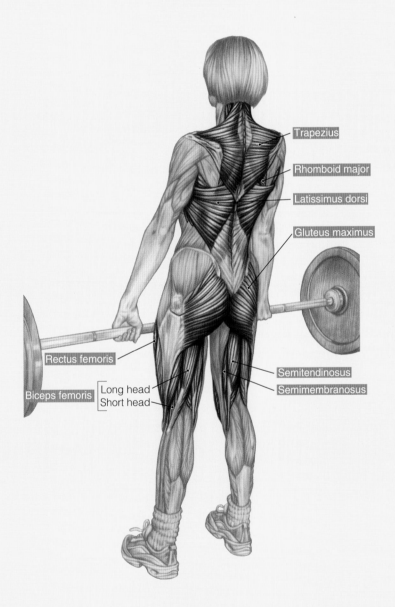

Trapezius

Rhomboid major

Latissimus dorsi

Gluteus maximus

Rectus femoris

Biceps femoris

Long head
Short head

Semitendinosus

Semimembranosus

Pro

- Because this exercise works so many muscles in very little time, it is one of the most complete and economical weight training exercises.

Cons

- The number of muscles this exercise recruits can make it very exhausting. Risks of accidents are high as a result of a poor mastering of technique or a loss of balance from fatigue.
- The deadlift may seem simple, but it is actually a very technical exercise. For this reason, you may want to avoid using it when you first start weightlifting.
- The deadlift may not be the best way to isolate and therefore specifically strengthen the lower back.[1] Furthermore, it is far riskier for the spine than isolating exercises such as the hyperextension performed on a bench (see the next exercise).

 The deadlift trains the lumbar muscles by putting a great deal of pressure on the spine. Make sure your spine remains aligned throughout the movement. After your workout, don't forget to decompress your spine by hanging from a pull-up bar for at least 20 to 30 seconds.

Tips

- To lift dumbbells or a barbell, do not pull with your legs first and then your back. Use them both at the same time.
- Curving your back to grab the weights (e.g., if you have long legs and short arms) puts your back in a bad position. If you can't reach the weights without curving your back, consider setting them on a bench a bit below knee level to reduce your range of motion.
- Keeping the slight natural arch in your back becomes more difficult as your lumbar muscles tire. At that point, your spine starts to curve. By arching your spine forward, you'll be able to handle heavier weight or push through a few more repetitions, which is why most women shift from a perfectly aligned back to a forward arch as the set progresses. However, this position places your back in a very hazardous position for the sake of a few more reps; the risk of injury is high, and we don't recommend this technique. Keep your back aligned even if it means you don't perform as many reps.

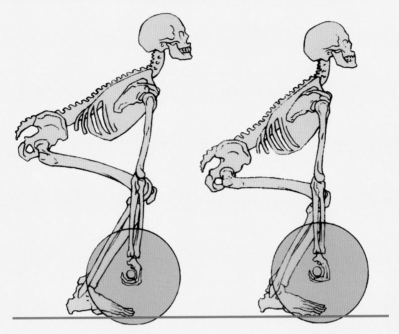

▌ Longer limbs (left) require more forward bend than short limbs (right).

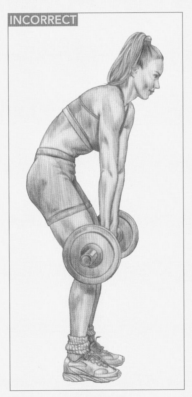

INCORRECT

▌ Stop the deadlift if you feel
your back start to curve.

243

Variations

- Bend your legs as you bring the weight down, or keep them almost straight during the whole movement. The latter increases the involvement of the hamstrings.

- Vary your foot placement by keeping your feet close together, which increases the range of motion. You will have to bend your back forward more, which will place more stress on your lumbar discs and muscles. On the other hand, spreading your feet wide apart (sumo position) reduces the range of motion, enabling you to keep your back straighter throughout the exercise.

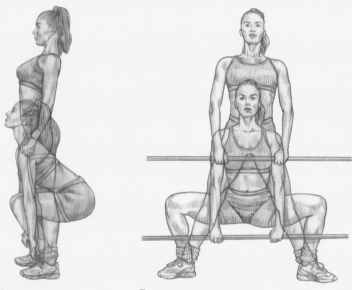

▌Narrow stance, greater range of motion

▌Wide stance, smaller range of motion

FREE WEIGHTS OR MACHINE?

Deadlift machines are increasingly more available. If you do not have access to one, you can perform the exercise on a Smith machine. The main difference between machines and free weights is that the movement is far easier on a machine because it is completely guided and you do not have to balance the bar. This lessens the chance of injuries due to a loss of balance as your muscles tire. Deteriorating technique as a result of fatigue is also less likely. Therefore, if you are a beginner, a machine is safer than free weights until you master the movement.

The hyperextension belongs in the isolating exercise category because only the hip joint is mobilized. Nevertheless, the hyperextension does recruit large muscle groups such as the lumbar muscles, the glutes, and the hamstrings. Unlike the deadlift, which tends to compress the intervertebral discs, the hyperextension is safer for the lower back but less effective in terms of overall strengthening. However, if your lower back is fragile, we recommend this isolating exercise over the deadlift.

How to Do It

Enter the bench, place your ankles under the padded brace, and bend over. Relax your spine for a second before slowly starting to raise your torso using your lumbar muscles. Once you are parallel to the floor (on a classic bench) or perpendicular to the floor (on a 45-degree bench), remain in the contracted position for a second before returning to the starting position and repeating.

▌ The movement

Semitendinosus

Semimembranosus

Gluteus maximus

Iliocostalis lumborum

Spinalis dorsi

Short head
Long head | Biceps femoris

Longissimus dorsi

Iliocostalis dorsi

▌ Hyperextension on a classic 90-degree bench

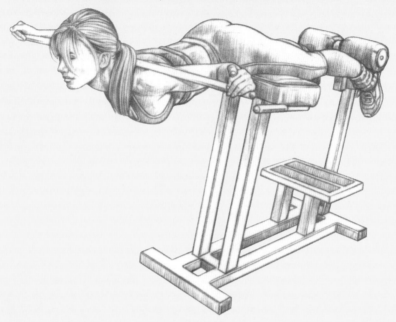

▌ **Increase the resistance by holding a bar or barbell on your shoulders.**

Pro

- The hyperextension is a safe way to strengthen the lumbar muscles, because, unlike the deadlift, it places very little tension on the intervertebral discs.

Con

- The movement becomes very easy very quickly, which reduces its effectiveness even if you try to overload the movement by holding a weight plate over your head or against your chest.

To avoid damaging your spine, perform the hyperextension in a slow, controlled manner. The lower back muscles are meant to contract more in an isometric manner rather than explosively. If you feel any pain in your spine on the way up, do not raise your back any higher.

Tip

- Placing the padded brace low over your quadriceps forces your glutes to provide most of the work, reducing the involvement of your lower back muscles. Placing the brace over your lower abs forces the lumbar muscles to provide most of the effort. As you can see, the hyperextension can become a lumbar or a glute exercise depending on where you place the brace that holds your torso.

Variations

Two main lower back benches are available.

- **90-degree bench:** As shown earlier, the classic bench places you parallel to the floor. This bench is not very comfortable to get into and use, but it provides more resistance for the lumbar muscles and a stronger stretch for the spine in the bottom position. It is therefore a more advanced bench.

- **45-degree bench:** Because of its inclination, this bench is easy to get into and out of. The resistance imposed by gravity is less than with a 90-degree bench, so it is easier to start with. However, the range of motion as well as the stretch of the spine is less than with a 90-degree bench. The 45-degree bench is a good choice if you are a beginner or cannot stand to have your head upside down.

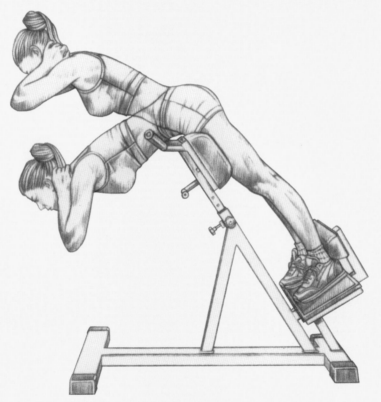

▌ **Hyperextension on a 45-degree inclined bench**

BENCH OR MACHINE?

With lower back machines, you have to bend over a great deal to get into position, which is uncomfortable. Furthermore, it is not easy to contract the lumbar muscles in a seated position. Therefore, we do not recommend these machines especially if back benches (also called Roman chairs) are available.

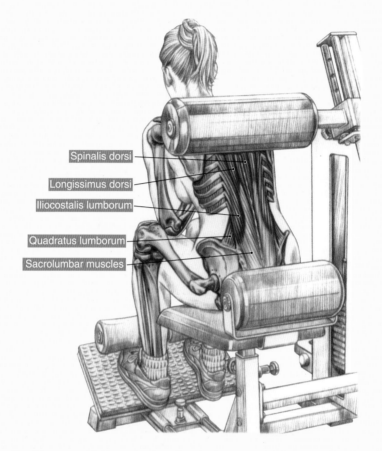

Spinalis dorsi

Longissimus dorsi

Iliocostalis lumborum

Quadratus lumborum

Sacrolumbar muscles

You'll see machines at the gym for the hyperextension exercise, but the position can be uncomfortable, and it is difficult to contract the lumbar muscles from this position.

- **Stretch after your workout:** Many weight training exercises compress the spine. To accelerate lumbar recuperation, at the end of *each* workout, decompress your spine by hanging from a pull-up bar for at least 30 seconds. You should do so even if you do not feel any lower back compression. If your discs remain tight, it is because your lower back muscles are continuing to contract. Over time, you will learn how to relax them.

To facilitate relaxation, do a set of abdominal crunches to complete exhaustion to temporarily fatigue your nervous system. This nervous failure will momentarily force every muscles in your body to relax (including the ones that support the spine). Then, go immediately to the pull-up bar and hang from it.

While hanging, relax your entire body as much as possible for at least 30 seconds. If your lower back remains tight, repeat this stretching procedure for several sets.

Hanging from a bar saves recovery time, because part of the spinal decompression that takes place during the night will already be done. The spine will recover faster, and you will sleep better.

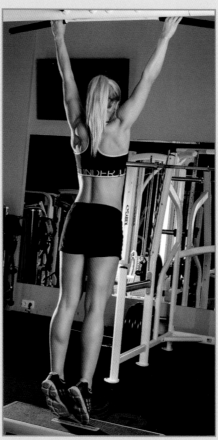

Hanging from a pull-up bar

- **Stretch on rest days:** Being upright and sitting down during the day also compress the spine. This compression squeezes out the fluid inside each disc, which is why people are shorter in the evening than they are in the morning. The fluid in your discs is indispensable for the health of your spine, and a loss of this fluid is at the heart of back pain. In theory, this lost fluid is replaced during the night while you sleep because lying down allows the spine to decompress.

  You may wake in the morning feeling as though your spine is still compressed. This means that the lumbar muscles have not relaxed enough. Because of nocturnal muscular tension, you have slept poorly, and you have not refilled your discs with their vital fluid. This could quickly translate to back pain.

  You can avoid this very common problem by relaxing your lumbar muscles and spine before going to sleep. Even on rest days, hang from a simple pull-up bar stuck in a doorway for 30 seconds just before you go to sleep.

Please, do not wait until you are suffering from back issues to take care of your spine. Prevention is the key. If you already suffer from back pain, consult your back specialist before engaging in weight training and practicing any back suspension.

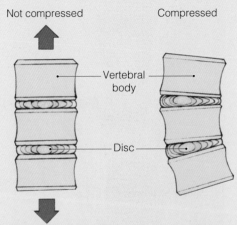

During exercise, the discs can become compressed (pinched in the front and bulging in the back). Hanging from a bar allows the vertebrae to move apart and reduces disc compression.

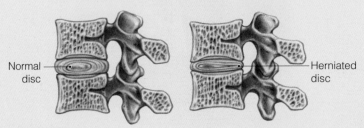

Too much disc compression can trigger a herniated disc.

Anatomy and Morphology

The pectoralis muscles allow you to move your arms forward when they must overcome a resistance (e.g., when pushing a door). They are also indispensable for keeping your arms together; for example, when holding a baby. In that case, the biceps are doing most of the work, but the chest muscles ensure that your arms remain close together. Without them, you would not be able to hold a baby very long.

The pectoralis major contains three heads:

1. The clavicular head, also known as the upper chest
2. The sternocostal head, which is the central part of the chest
3. The abdominal head, which is the lower chest

The pectoralis minor is a very small muscle hidden under the pectoralis muscles. As the name implies, it is of very minor importance.

The pectoralis muscles are often underdeveloped because they are generally not used in everyday activities. Thus, they are not muscles that feel natural to contract.

The chest muscle is a single-joint muscle because it crosses only the shoulder joint. On the other hand, because of its fanlike shape, it is an angled muscle. This means that you can work this muscle from many angles: an inclined, flat, or declined position.

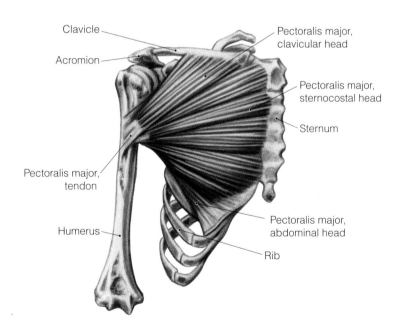

Clavicle
Acromion
Pectoralis major, clavicular head
Pectoralis major, sternocostal head
Sternum
Pectoralis major, tendon
Pectoralis major, abdominal head
Humerus
Rib

251

The goals of this warm-up sequence are to prepare the following muscles for training and reduce the risk of injury:

- Tendon of the long head of the biceps
- Shoulder, elbow, and wrist joints
- Chest muscles and tendons
- Triceps

Perform 20 to 30 easy repetitions of the following exercises using light weights. Move from one exercise to the next without any rest. If you do not feel that one cycle has warmed you up, feel free to perform a second cycle.

Once you have finished this overall warm-up cycle, move on to the chest press using at least two light sets to specifically warm up your chest before handling heavier weights. If you are already warmed up because you have just finished training your back or your shoulders, there is no need to repeat this entire warm-up sequence. However, you should still do two sets of a specific chest exercise as a warm-up.

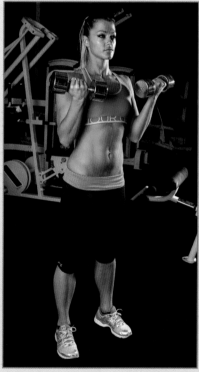

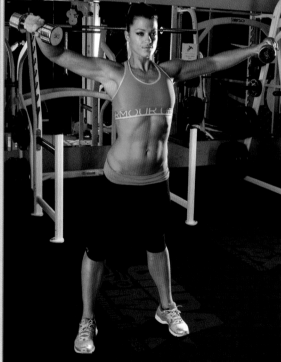

1. Biceps curl (see page 276)   **2. Lateral raise (see page 196)**

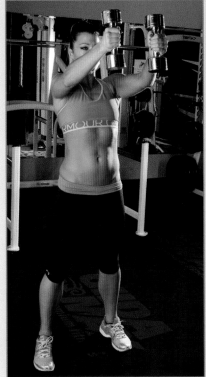

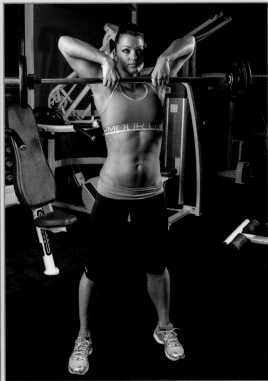

3. Front raise (see page 205)

4. Upright row (see page 206)

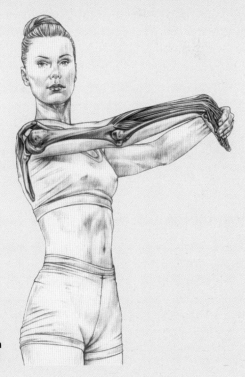

5. Wrist stretch
(see page 304)

The chest press belongs in the basic, multiple-joint exercise category because both the shoulder and the elbow joints are mobilized. As a result, the press recruits many muscle groups in addition to the chest: the front area of the shoulders, the triceps, and the upper part of the back.

The press is considered a good starting exercise because it stimulates so many muscles of the upper body. Because of this diversity of muscle recruitment, people can handle a significant amount of weight.

How to Do It

Lie with your back on a bench or the seat of a machine. Grab the barbell, dumbbells, or handles. If you are using dumbbells, bring them to your shoulders with a pronated grip (thumbs toward each other). Straighten your arms using your chest muscles. Dumbbells should touch at the height of the movement. Then, lower the weight by bending your arms.

Pro

- Because it stimulates a large amount of muscle mass in a very short time, the press can be the cornerstone of your upper-body training.

Con

- It is easy to lose control of the load, especially with free weights. You are likely to get hurt if the weight falls on you. If possible, start by using machines instead of free weights until you master the proper pressing techniques. After a few weeks of machine training, you can switch to free weights if you so desire.

Dumbbells require special attention to ensure safety. To protect your back when lifting them from the floor to your starting position, first place them on your thighs with your arms bent. When laying them down, be careful not to stretch your arms and drop them, because doing so could tear your biceps.

FREE WEIGHTS OR MACHINE?

The chest press can be performed with free weights (barbell or dumbbells) or a machine. Analyze the advantages and disadvantages of each version to choose the one that suits you best.

Pro of Barbell Presses

- You can bench press in every gym or even at home with a simple barbell and a bench. However, despite the ready availability of the equipment, using a barbell has more drawbacks than advantages.

Cons of Barbell Presses

- Balancing a long barbell is not easy and might even prove dangerous for beginners.
- Unracking the barbell and replacing it are hazardous for the joints; these movements offer no muscle-strengthening effects.
- The barbell may fall on you at the end of a set when your muscle strength suddenly diminishes.
- For all these reasons, a training partner is required.

▌ Start position

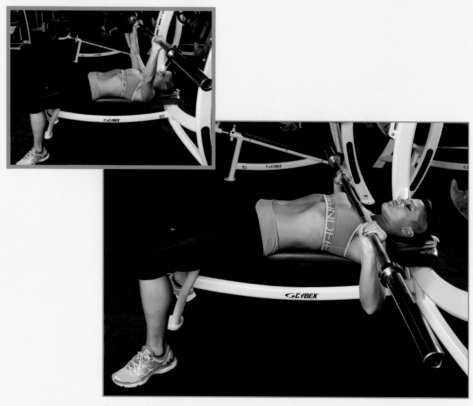

▌ Barbell press

Pros of Dumbbell Presses

- The degree of contraction is far greater with dumbbells than with a barbell because in the contracted position your hands end up closer together.
- You can adopt any hand and elbow position. This freedom is much more restricted with a barbell.

Con of Dumbbell Presses

- Balancing dumbbells is not easy and might even prove dangerous if you let one go during the last repetition of a set as your strength lessens. This is most common with beginners.

▌ **Start position**

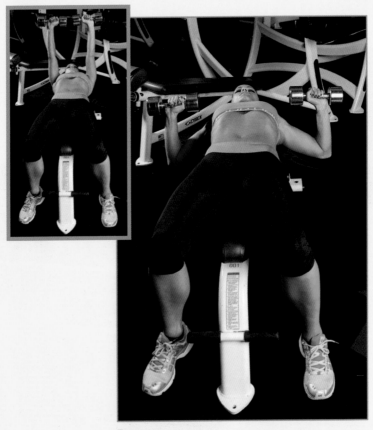

▌ **Dumbbell press**

Pros of Smith Machine Presses

- A Smith machine can be a good compromise between a barbell and a machine, yet safer than free weights for a beginner. The advantage of a Smith machine is that you do not have to balance the weight, which reduces the need for a partner.
- Safety pins are available on every good Smith machine. In the case of a sudden loss of strength, the bar will crash on them rather than on you. Therefore, do not forget to put them on!

Con of Smith Machine Presses

- The movement involves a potentially dangerous (for some women's morphology), unnatural linear trajectory rather than a slightly circular arc, as it does with free weights and with most good machines.

▌ Start position

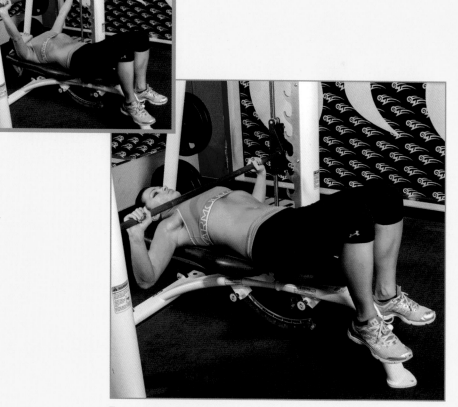

▌ Smith machine press

Pros of Machine Presses

- If you are a beginner, you may have difficulty pressing while lying on a bench. It may even feel very unnatural to be forced to mobilize all your strength in that position. In that case, machines that allow you to press while seated may be better suited for you.
- Machines are very stable and do not require you to balance the weight.
- No manipulation of the barbell or dumbbells is required. Everything is already in place. You need only press, concentrating strictly on your chest muscles.
- Overall, good machines are much safer and easier to use than free weights, especially if you are new to fitness.

Con of Machine Presses

- There are more poorly designed machines than there are good ones. As a beginner, it is hard to know which ones are good and which ones are bad. As a rule of thumb, with the best machines, you bring your hands closer together as you press the weight; as you bring the weight down, your hands get farther apart. A good machine duplicates the range of motion of dumbbells without the constraint of having to balance the load.

Variations in Bench Angle

The three main variations of the press are performed as follows:

1. On a flat bench, to recruit the whole chest muscle
2. On an incline bench, to favor the recruitment of the upper part of the chest
3. On a decline bench, to better target the lower chest

Machines also offer these variations, although because you are seated, they may not be apparent. How you are pushing on the machine indicates the variation as follows:

1. Pushing up duplicates the motion of an incline bench.
2. Pushing out in front of you targets the whole chest just as a flat bench does.
3. Pushing down mimics the motion on a decline bench.

For women, using an incline bench or a machine that duplicates it is most appropriate because this version recruits more of the upper part of the chest as well as the front shoulders. As mentioned earlier, it is far more useful for women to work the visible part of the chest. Furthermore, because the front shoulder receives enough indirect work from this exercise, you do not have to train it separately. Therefore, the incline press is most effective and saves time as well. Note that because the effort is more localized in the upper chest area rather than in the overall pectoral, you cannot handle as heavy a weight with the incline press as you can with a flat or decline press.

The declined position is useful only for men who want to accentuate the separation of the chest from the upper abs. It has no utility for women.

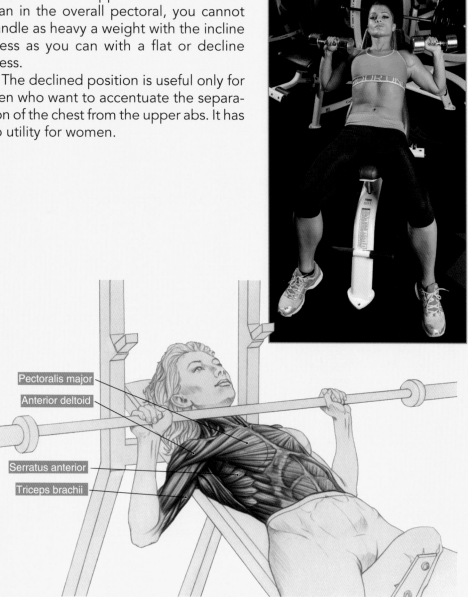

▍ **Dumbbell press on an incline bench**

Pectoralis major
Anterior deltoid
Serratus anterior
Triceps brachii

▍ **Barbell press on an incline bench**

Variations in Where the Bar Is Lowered

The ending point of the movement should be determined based on your goal:

- Bringing the bar to the upper chest level works the upper part of the pectoralis muscle more than the lower. This is ideal if you train on an incline bench.
- Bringing the bar to the lower part of the chest works the lower part of the pectoralis more than the upper. This is ideal if you train on a flat or decline bench.

Variations in Hand and Elbow Position

With dumbbells and with some machines, the orientation of the hands and the elbows can vary. Consider the following variations to determine which works your chest the way you like, and the most safely.

- To stretch the pectoralis major less and work the shoulders more, keep your elbows alongside your body and your hands in a neutral position (thumbs toward your head).
- To stretch the chest muscles at the bottom of the movement and work your pectoralis muscle harder, spread your elbows as far from your body as possible and use a pronated grip (thumbs facing each other). Be aware, however, that this position puts you at greater risk of tearing the tendon of your chest.

Variations in Grip Width

- **Wide grip:** The farther apart your hands are at the bottom part of the press, the more you stretch the chest muscles. Not all of your tendons will appreciate this stretch, especially if you have long forearms. Furthermore, once your arms are straight, the contraction shortens the chest muscles to a lesser degree.
- **Narrow grip:** The closer together your hands are at the bottom part of the press, the less stretch there is on the chest. This is less risky for the pectoralis tendon. There is a greater shortening of the pectoralis muscles once the arm is straight. The only drawback is that the triceps, which are recruited more with the narrow grip, take over some of the work from the pectoralis muscles.

Overall, it is wise to avoid the extremely wide grip used in strength competitions to reduce the range of motion and permit the handling of heavier weights. A slightly narrower grip than normal is the safest position as long as it does not irritate your elbow joints.

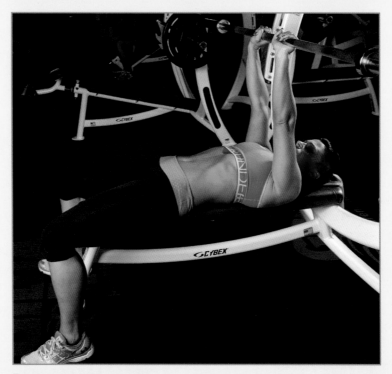

▌ **Press with a narrow grip**

Tips

- Arching your lower back reduces the range of motion, allowing you to handle heavier weights. However, it makes you more prone to back injuries and transfers the muscular tension from the upper to the lower part of the chest, rendering the exercise less productive. Arching the back might be a good strategy for men, but not for women.

- Do not move your head from side to side or up and down while pressing. Keep it safely on the bench to avoid any shaking movement of the neck.

- The bench press is like a reverse push-up. Instead of moving your body, you move only your arms. If you do not have access to weightlifting equipment, push-ups are a good alternative.

The chest fly belongs in the isolating exercise category because only the shoulder joint is mobilized. As a consequence, the fly does not recruit much of the muscle groups surrounding the chest. Unlike the press, which also stimulates the triceps, the fly only indirectly works the front part of the shoulders in addition to the chest, its main target. The fly is considered a good finishing chest exercise because of this muscular isolation, as well as the nice stretch it provides.

How to Do It: Dumbbell Fly

Grab two dumbbells, sit on the edge of the bench, and bring the dumbbells to your shoulders using a neutral hand grip (thumbs pointing up) as you lower your back onto the bench. Straighten your arms in front of you as if you were doing a bench press.

Once in position, lower your arms to your sides while keeping them semi-straight. When your hands are at about the same level as your chest, bring the dumbbells together using your chest muscles. Then, lower the weights again by moving the dumbbells apart without bending your arms too much.

▌ Start position

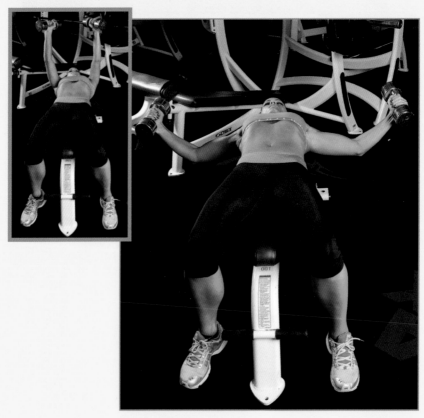

▌ Dumbbell fly

The dumbbells do not have to touch at the top of the movement. In fact, there is little resistance at the height of the exercise. If you cannot feel your chest muscles when your arms are up, it is better to work under continuous tension. To avoid losing the contraction in your chest muscle, stop the dumbbells at three quarters of the movement rather than perform it completely.

With dumbbells, you can rotate your wrists to feel the pectoralis muscles contracting more. In one version, the closer your hands are together, the more you will turn your pinkie fingers toward each other. The contraction will be more pronounced in the lower pectoralis muscles. In a second version, the closer your hands are together, the more you will turn your thumbs toward each other. The contraction will be more pronounced in the upper pectoralis muscles and shoulders.

FREE WEIGHTS OR MACHINE?

During a free-weight fly, the resistance is very uneven over the range of motion. The tension is very high in the stretched position, which increases the risk of overstretching the tendons of both the chest and the long head of the biceps. As you bring the weights up, the resistance decreases dramatically. It is almost null at the top of the movement. Studies estimate that the resistance on the chest muscles is insignificant over more than 25 percent of this exercise.[1]

The machine fly avoids these limitations because good machines do the following:

- Provide a gentler stretch of the chest muscles in the bottom position.
- Keep more tension in the contracting phase of the movement.

Therefore, it is wiser and safer to use a machine rather than dumbbells. If you do not have access to a machine, you can perform the fly on a cable crossover machine.

How to Do It: Machine Fly

Sit in the machine and grab one pad or handle, and then the other. Bring the two pads or handles together until they touch. Remain in this contracted position for one second and bring your arms back. Unlike with dumbbells, make sure you bring your hands as close as possible to really squeeze the chest muscles. Do not overstretch your chest in the starting position.

▌ Machine fly

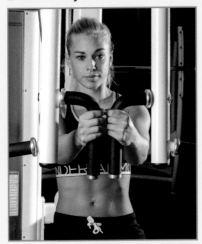

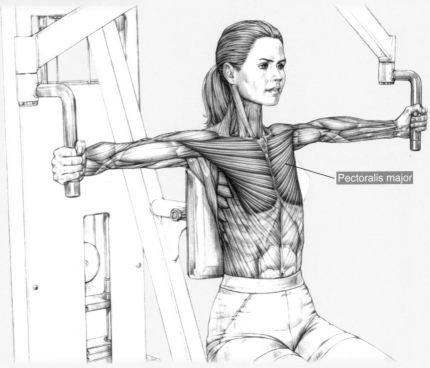

Pectoralis major

▌ Start position

How to Do It: Cable Crossover

Grab one handle and then the other with your arms parallel to the floor, forming a T with your body. Then bring your arms in toward your body. Remain in this contracted position for one second and bring your arms back up (you can also cross your arms as shown to increase the range of motion). The main advantage of the cable over dumbbells or a machine is that you can bring your arms either toward your abdomen or toward your head (or anywhere else between these two points) to change the angle at which the pectoralis muscles work. In fact, the chest area should be worked at a variety of angles.

The lower you bring your arms down, the more you'll target your lower chest. A higher arm position at the shoulder or head level stimulates the upper portion of the chest more. As noted earlier, from an aesthetic standpoint, women typically don't need to train the lower part of the chest intensely; the upper chest is more important.

▌ **Start position**

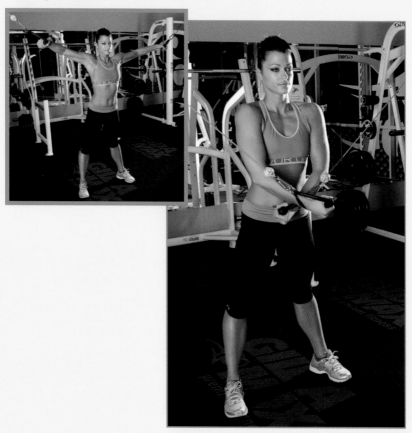

▌ **Cable crossover**

Start position

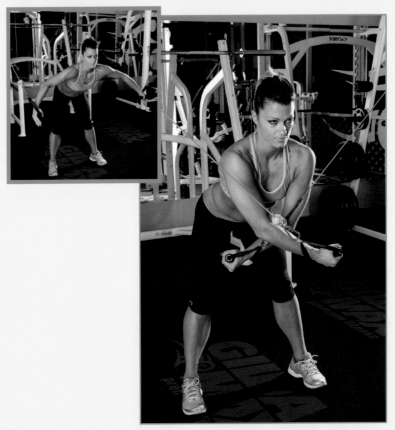

The bent-over cable crossover variation targets the mid-chest region

Pros

- The chest fly provides a good stretch for the pectoralis muscles.
- Unlike with the bench press, the triceps muscles are not involved, which means they will not tire before the pectoralis muscles do.

Cons

- It can be difficult to focus the contraction on the pectoralis muscles only and not on the shoulders.
- Because almost no resistance exists at the top of the movement, it can be difficult to feel the pectoralis muscles contract when using dumbbells.

Never straighten your arms completely during the exercise because doing so places too much unwanted stress on the biceps tendons.

Tips

- To really stimulate your chest muscles, you must do this exercise slowly and with continuous tension. Avoid any jerking of the weights.

- If you have trouble feeling your pectoralis muscles during multiple-joint exercises such as the press, you can learn to feel their contractions using the fly. After a few weeks of training with this isolating movement, you will have better sensations during the basic pectoralis exercises.

- With dumbbells or with the cable crossover, the exercise is much easier if you bend your arms; this is why you should make an effort not to bend your arms more and more as the set goes on. When you reach failure, you can always bend your arms a little so that you can perform a few more repetitions. The same problem occurs on machines, which have you perform the fly with your arms in a semistraight position.

- With machines that have you do the fly with your arms bent, the main mistake is to push with your hands, which forces the elbows to leave the pad. On such machines, make sure you are pushing with your elbows rather than with your hands to keep the tension on your chest muscles.

Variations

As with the press, there are three main variations of the dumbbell fly, which are performed as follows:

1. On a flat bench, to recruit the whole chest muscle

2. On an incline bench, to favor the recruitment of the upper part of the chest

3. On a decline bench, to isolate the lower chest

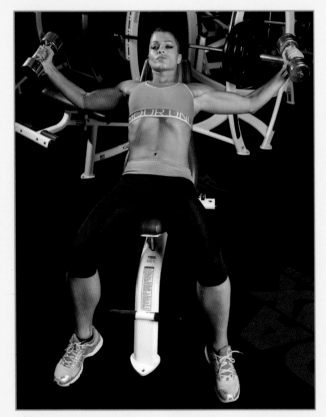

▌ **Dumbbell fly on an incline bench**

The pullover belongs in the isolated, single-joint exercise category because only the shoulder joint is mobilized. Even though the chest, the latissimus dorsi, and the triceps muscles are recruited, the pullover should not be considered a muscle-building exercise for the chest. Rather, use it to stretch your shoulders and rib cage to improve your posture.

How to Do It

Grab a dumbbell, holding it with both hands in a neutral grip (thumbs toward your head). Lie on your back either completely on the bench or across the bench.

Your head should be just on the edge of the bench so that your arms can hang freely over it. This will provide a greater range of motion and a better stretch. If you are lying across the bench, your shoulders should be just on the edge of the bench to avoid any excessive stretch.

Once in position, straighten your arms above your head. Take a deep breath so that you inflate your rib cage to its maximum, and try to squeeze your shoulder blades together. You should feel your rib cage opening up. While keeping your arms in a semistraight position, lower the weight behind your head.

When your arms are extended from your body, raise them back up using the strength of your pectoralis muscles while exhaling all the air so that you deflate your rib cage. Stop the movement when the dumbbell is above your head, and then lower it again.

With the across-the-bench pullover, lower your buttocks in parallel with your hands to accentuate the stretching effect. As you raise your hands, raise your buttocks simultaneously.

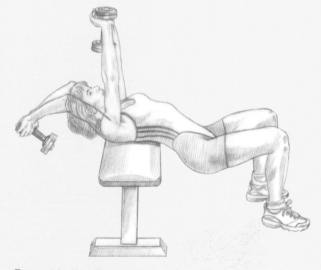

▌ **Dumbbell pullover across a bench**

FREE WEIGHTS OR MACHINE?

Machine pullovers are designed to work on the lats and chest muscles rather than to stretch the rib cage. For purposes of developing the chest, it is best to stick to free weights.

Pros

- The pullover stretches the pectoralis muscles and shoulders simultaneously (two groups that tend to naturally lack flexibility).
- It helps increase endurance because of the respiratory muscle work it provides.

Con

- The pullover places the shoulder joints in a relatively unstable position. For this reason, avoid using a weight that's too heavy. Increase the number of repetitions rather than the weight. Try to feel the stretch rather than anything else.

 Avoid this exercise if you suffer from any shoulder pain or injury.

Tips

- You can bend your arms very slightly to increase the stretch, but if you bend them too much, the work will transfer to the back muscles, robbing the effort from the pectoralis muscles.
- Don't bring the dumbbell all the way back down to your abdomen; stop it when it is above your head. With free weights, the more you bring your arms up, the less resistance you place on your muscles. Therefore, it is best to use a limited range of motion by not raising your arms too high past your head.

Variations

- Pullovers can be performed with either a dumbbell or a barbell. The latter places more unwanted stress on the shoulder joints because it is far harder to balance. Therefore, the dumbbell pullover is the better choice.
- Pullovers can be performed while lying on a bench or across a bench. The latter version provides a much greater stretch. If you are a beginner, you can start by lying on the bench, especially if you lack flexibility. Once you feel comfortable with this version, shift to the more advanced variation of lying across the bench.

STRETCH THE CHEST

It is very important to stretch the chest muscles because they tend to lack flexibility, which brings the shoulders forward. This position results in poor posture and contributes to damaging the upper part of the spine by rounding the back.

- **Bilateral chest stretch:** Clasp both hands behind your back and slowly lift them away from your body. Although stretching both arms at the same time is possible, doing so reduces the range of motion. Stretch both arms at the same time during your first month of training. After this, begin doing the unilateral version.

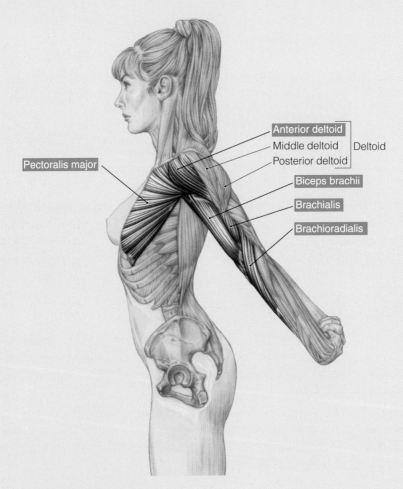

Pectoralis major

Anterior deltoid

Middle deltoid — Deltoid

Posterior deltoid

Biceps brachii

Brachialis

Brachioradialis

▍ Bilateral chest stretch

- **Unilateral chest stretch:** Stand in a doorway or beside a squat rack. Place your left arm, bent to 90 degrees, against the frame. Support yourself against the frame using your hand and elbow. Take a small step forward and lean forward. Hold the stretched position for 10 to 30 seconds before returning your arms to the starting position. Once you are finished stretching the left/right pectoralis, move on to your left arm. When stretching with your arm bent becomes too easy, straighten it more to accentuate the difficulty of the exercise as shown.

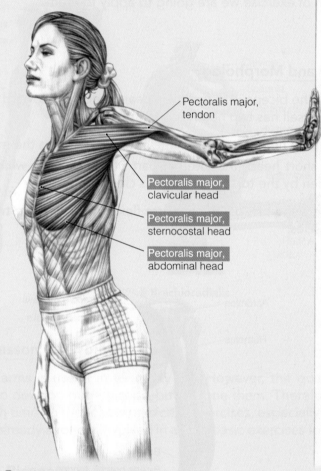

Pectoralis major, tendon

Pectoralis major, clavicular head

Pectoralis major, sternocostal head

Pectoralis major, abdominal head

▌ Unilateral chest stretch

CURL

Pro

- With dumbbell curls, your arms are free to use the most natural path possible for your anatomy.

Con

- Because the temptation to cheat is stronger in this exercise than any other, many people do not really work the biceps.

- **You can use a heavier weight or do a few more repetitions if you swing your torso from front to back. However, doing so increases the risk of injuring your back. To learn to do the exercise perfectly, begin by doing it with your back against a wall to keep your torso from moving.**
- **During all biceps exercises performed in supination, do not completely straighten your arms in the lengthened position. In that position, the biceps is susceptible to tearing. This is especially true for women, because most of them have a greater range of motion in the biceps than men because of an anatomical particularity called a recurvatum at the elbow level (see page 291 for more information). Most women can overextend their arms if they want to. Their forearms do not stop when in a straight line with their upper arms, as most men's do. Women can bring their forearms back farther, which stretches the biceps, placing it in a precarious situation in case it should contract powerfully. We strongly recommend that you do not use this extra range of motion during any form of curl (as well as during the back exercises). It is much safer to keep constant tension in the biceps by stopping the exercise a little before your arms are completely straight.**

Tips

- We recommend that you do not perform several forms of curls during the same workout. If you like variety, alternate by doing classic supinated curls during one workout and a different form of curl in the next workout.
- If you suffer from back pain, you can perform biceps curls safely by using a low pulley. Instead of standing, lie on the floor to perform your curls. In that position, very little tension is placed on your spine and your back remains in a perfectly straight position with no possibility of swinging.

Supinated Curl

How to Do It

Grasp a dumbbell in each hand using a supinated hand position. Use your biceps to bend your arm. Bring the weight as high as possible and hold at the top, contracted position for one second while squeezing your forearm tightly against your biceps. Now lower the weight slowly back to your start position. Repeat with the other arm. Another option is to lift both dumbbells at once. Lifting both arms simultaneously saves you time and forces you to work on your balance. On the other hand, alternating arms allows you to lift slightly more weight or do more repetitions with the same weight because one arm is provided extra rest time while you flex the other. You can also start with your hands in a neutral position with the thumbs facing forward. In this case, rotate the wrist to bring your thumb toward the outside as you bend your arm.

▌ Start position

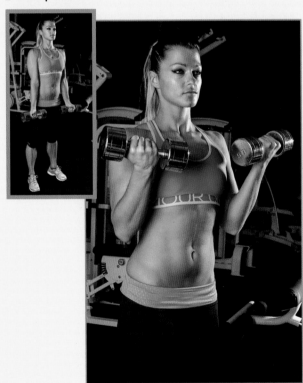

▌ Supinated bilateral dumbbell curl

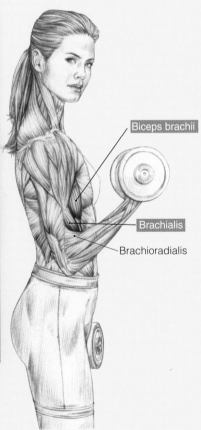

Biceps brachii

Brachialis

Brachioradialis

▌ Supinated unilateral dumbbell curl

Tips

- Keep your hand supinated throughout the set or rotate your wrist with every repetition, whichever feels most natural. If you choose supination throughout the movement, do not straighten your arm completely at the bottom of the movement, especially with heavy weights, to avoid tearing your biceps muscle. To avoid this risk altogether, keep your hand neutral in the outstretched position.
- Don't lift your elbows up when raising the dumbbells. You may lift the elbow slightly but do not lift it in an exaggerated fashion.

Variations

- You can do dumbbell curls either sitting or standing. It's easier to maintain proper form while sitting, so one strategy is to begin the exercise seated. At failure, stand up so that you can do a few more repetitions by cheating on your form a little.
- You can use a long bar instead of a dumbbell as long as the movement feels natural. If it does not, try an EZ bar instead of a straight bar because it is gentler on the joints, especially the wrist. You can also perform the curl with an attachment on a low pulley, but note that a pulley with a long bar has the same disadvantages as training with a barbell, so consider other attachments, like a V-bar. However, we believe that dumbbells are ideal for biceps exercises (one-arm cable curls will provide the same benefits as dumbbells).

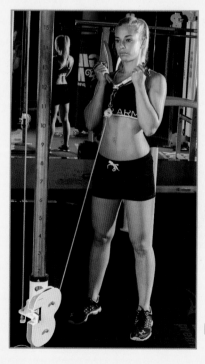

▌ **Supinated curl at a low pulley using a V bar**

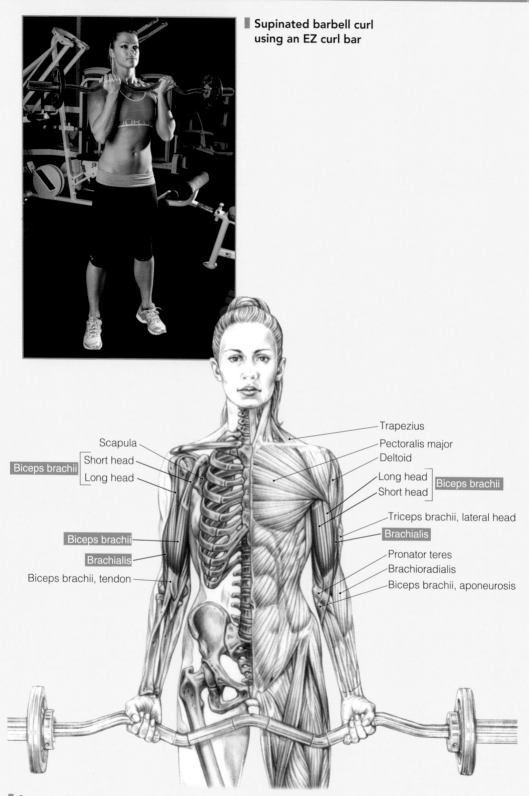

Supinated barbell curl using an EZ curl bar

Scapula

Biceps brachii
Short head
Long head

Biceps brachii

Brachialis

Biceps brachii, tendon

Trapezius
Pectoralis major
Deltoid

Long head
Short head
Biceps brachii

Triceps brachii, lateral head

Brachialis

Pronator teres
Brachioradialis
Biceps brachii, aponeurosis

Start position

FREE WEIGHTS OR MACHINE?

The biceps curl machine shown here provides far more freedom of movement than most; biceps machines are generally poorly designed, especially for women. Men's arms tend to be relatively straight, whereas women's arms are usually bent more at the elbow level. This anatomical bend is called a valgus. Because women's hips tend to be larger than men's, this valgus is very useful because it allows the arms to hang freely at the sides without bumping into the iliac crests all the time.

Very few machine manufacturers have taken this major morphological difference between men and women into account. This is why most biceps machines feel so weird to women: The movement arms want to bring your hands down in a straight line while your forearms want to go toward the outside. There is nothing wrong with this feeling, and there is nothing wrong with you. The problem lies with the design of the machine. In time, this movement will result in injury. Free weights, especially dumbbells, are much better than machines because you bring them along the natural path of your arm and not the other way around.

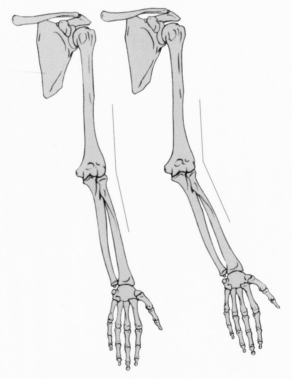

The arm on the left is relatively straight, whereas the arm on the right is bent at the elbow.

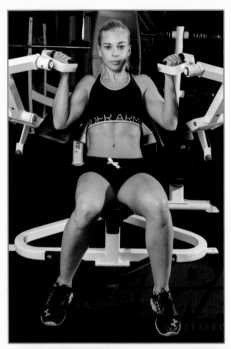

Bilateral machine curl

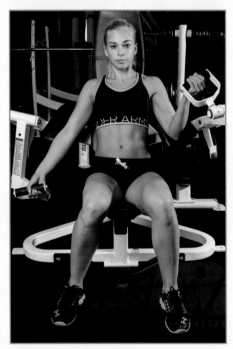

Unilateral machine curl

Hammer Curl

How to Do It

Hold two dumbbells in a neutral position (thumbs up) during the whole set. As opposed to supinated curls, which really target the biceps, this isolation exercise specifically targets the brachialis and brachioradialis muscles and does not stimulate the biceps as much. We show here hammer curls with dumbbells, a low pulley, and weight plates. All three versions are very similar as far as their muscle focus; try them all to discover which one is the most comfortable and works the best for you.

▌ **Start position**

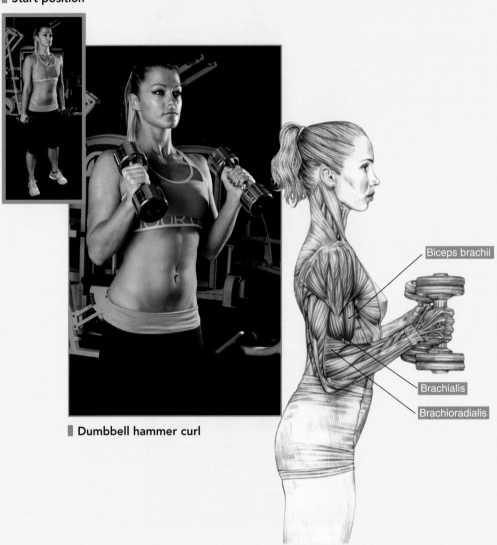

▌ **Dumbbell hammer curl**

Biceps brachii

Brachialis

Brachioradialis

Tip

- Your arm is stronger when you use a neutral, rather than a supinated, hand position. For this reason, you can use heavier weights with hammer curls than with classic supinated curls. Just be careful that the weight doesn't result in a reduced range of motion.

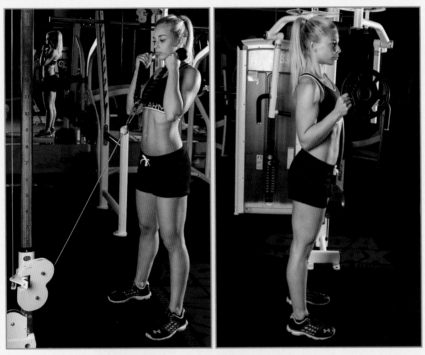

Hammer curl at a low pulley   Hammer curl using weight plates

Reverse Curl

How to Do It

Hold two dumbbells or a bar using a pronated hand position (palms down with the thumbs facing each other) during the whole set. This isolation exercise specifically targets the brachioradialis, the brachialis, and a little bit of the biceps.

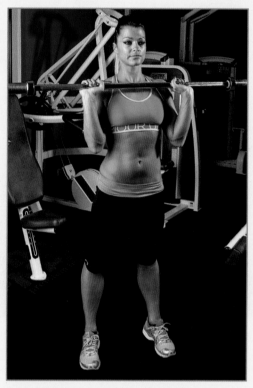

▌ **Reverse curl using a straight bar**

Tip

- If you feel that a straight bar places too much stress on your wrists, try using an EZ bar instead. If you still feel an unnatural twist of your forearms, dumbbells are the solution. In that case, instead of having both thumbs facing each other, bring them up slightly so that you minimize the rotation of your hands.

Curl With the Elbows Elevated

How to Do It

When your elbow is elevated, the brachialis muscle works a bit more and the biceps a bit less than with classic (supinated) curls. This particularly emphasizes the interior of the biceps. It is what happens with the dumbbell concentration curl, with the preacher curl on a Larry Scott bench, and on most machines.

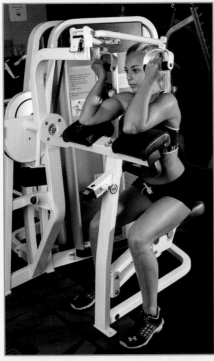

▌ Seated machine curl with elbows elevated

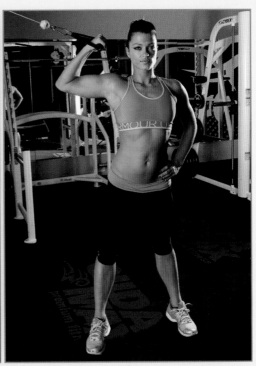

▌ Standing unilateral high-pulley curl with elbow elevated

Tip

- Straightening the arms completely is even more dangerous with the elbows elevated than with regular curls. Even if you see many people at the gym doing the exercise using a full stretch, shortening your range of motion will minimize the risk of tearing your biceps tendons.

Curl With the Elbows Behind the Body

How to Do It

Whenever you place your elbow behind your body (as during curls performed on an incline bench), you better isolate the exterior of the biceps. The interior head and the brachialis receive less stimulation.

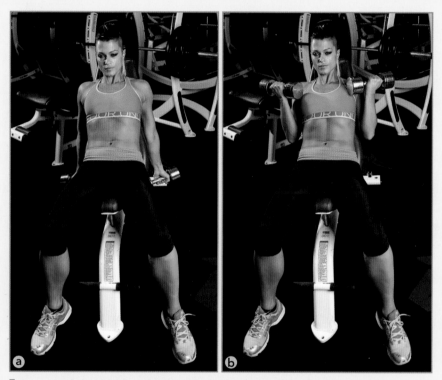

▮ Supinated dumbbell curl with the elbows behind the body

Tip

- If you feel an overwhelming stretch at the shoulder level, it means your arms are too far behind your body, a position that could damage the long head of the biceps tendon. This risk comes from using too flat of a bench; adjust it up closer to the 90° position instead.

Triceps

Anatomy and Morphology

The triceps has three heads. The lateral head (on the exterior) is the most visible. The other two heads are somewhat hidden by the torso. Therefore, you should focus on developing the lateral head so you can quickly see the results of your training. The triceps is the antagonistic muscle to the biceps and the brachialis. It extends the arm.

The long head of the triceps is the only one of the three heads of the triceps that is a multiple-joint muscle. It does more than just extend the arm as the other two heads do; it also helps bring the arm toward the body or to the rear, in conjunction with the back and rear shoulder muscles. As such, it is involved in all back and rear shoulder exercises. For this reason, to avoid the all-too-common elbow injuries, carefully warm up your elbows before working your back.

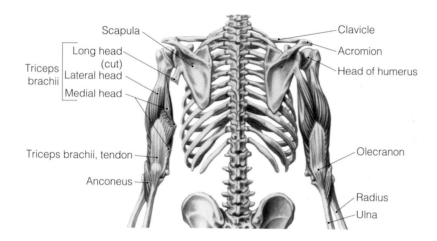

Take-Home Lesson for Women

As with the biceps, most women do not strive to develop huge triceps. Simply toning them a little is a common goal. The main difference between biceps and triceps is that the back of the arm is an important storage area for fat in women. By training your triceps frequently with lighter weight and high repetitions, you can prevent this deposit of fat.

Triceps training is important not only for immediate results but also for the future: After menopause, many women lose the fat covering the triceps as a result of hormonal disruptions. This shift can leave an excess of skin hanging from your arms. Once this sagging skin is in place, there is not much you can do to get rid of it except through surgery. This is why it is important to prevent the accumulation of fat on your triceps early in life.

Warm Up the Triceps

The great majority of women aren't looking to develop their triceps to be as large as a man's and thus don't start the workout with the arms, so there is no need to repeat a triceps-specific warm-up sequence. You should still, however, perform at least one light set of the specific triceps exercise you are going to perform, as a warm-up.

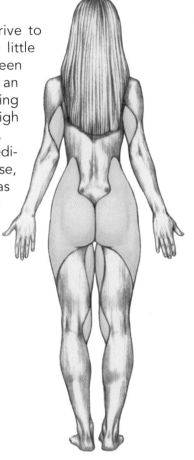

❚ The triceps is a natural fat storage area in women, more so than in men.

Triceps Exercises

There are four main categories of exercises for the triceps from which women can benefit:

1. Cable push-down
2. Triceps extension
3. Triceps kickback
4. Narrow grip press (this was described in the chest section on page 262)

Each category has several versions, which guarantees a great variety of movements and allows you to choose the ones that best suit both your anatomy and your goals.

Protect Your Elbow Joints

The elbow joint is very fragile. This is why we recommend avoiding using heavy weights for the direct triceps exercises. High repetitions with lighter weights are safer for the elbows. This strategy is also more in tune with your primary goal of keeping fat off your triceps.

The elbow joint is especially fragile in women as a result of their much greater range of forearm motion than men. Women's much more pronounced recurvatum at the elbow allows them to bring their forearms farther back than men can. This enhances the contraction of the triceps, but it also places the elbow joint in a very vulnerable position. If you are using heavy weights in any triceps exercises or in the chest or shoulder presses, do not straighten your arms completely to avoid placing your elbow joints in this precarious position.

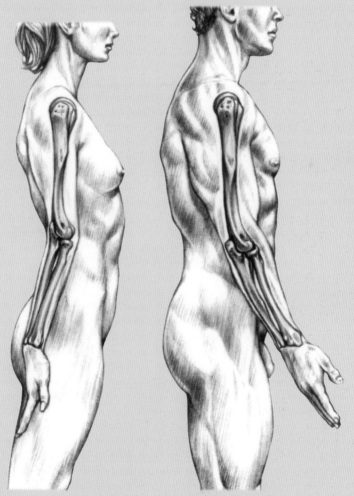

Women possess a much more pronounced recurvatum at the elbow than men.

CABLE PUSH-DOWN

The push-down belongs in the isolating exercise category because only the elbow joint is mobilized. As a result, the push-down does not recruit many muscles except the triceps and the forearm flexors.

How to Do It

Attach a short triceps bar, straight bar, or rope to the upper part of a pulley machine. You can grab the rope with your hands in a neutral position (thumbs pointing up), the triceps bar in a semineutral or pronated position (thumbs facing each other), and the straight bar in a pronated position. Use whichever grip allows you to contract your triceps the most.

Push on the bar or rope so that you bring your hands to your thighs while keeping your elbows close to your sides. Hold the contracted position for one second before returning to the starting position without moving your elbows. You can stand with your feet together, or staggered; the staggered stance shown here is more challenging to your balance.

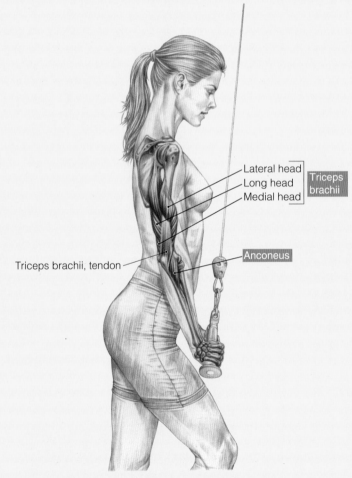

Lateral head
Long head
Medial head
Triceps brachii

Anconeus

Triceps brachii, tendon

▌ Push-down using a triceps bar and pronated grip

Start position

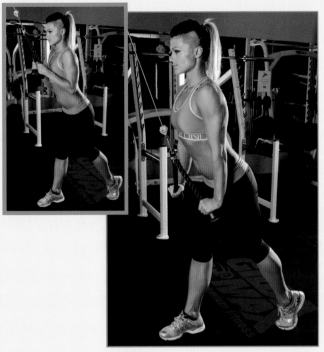

Push-down using a rope attachment and neutral grip

Start position

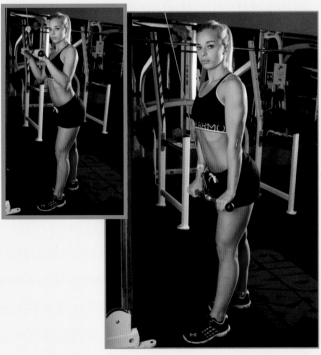

Push-down using a straight bar and pronated grip

CABLE PUSH-DOWN

Pro

- Working the triceps with a pulley is less traumatic for the elbow joints than using your body weight (as in doing push-ups), dumbbells, a barbell, or any other kind of machines. A more complex pulley network reduces the forces and thus is gentler for the joints.

Con

- Because the triceps is not used on a daily basis, many beginners have trouble feeling this muscle working. At first, do this exercise slowly so that you can learn to feel your triceps contracting.

- **Excessive weight can force your torso to move up, which will arch your spine as your hands are brought up. Limit this arch as much as possible and avoid any swaying of the torso.**
- **If you feel any pain in your elbows as you extend your forearms, do not completely lock your arms because full extension may be damaging for some women. Instead, use continuous tension by stopping short of complete extension.**

Tip

- Lifting your elbows while the bar is moving up is perceived as a mistake. This is true if you are trying to isolate your triceps. However, to work the triceps and the back in synergy as nature intended, you can lift your elbows to your chin or nose level while the bar is rising. Both your hands and your elbows will be pushed down as you press the bar. Many people in the gym are likely to comment that this technique is a mistake, but this only reveals their lack of anatomy knowledge. Do not let these people influence you.

Variation

- You have a choice as to how wide to place your hands on the bar. However, avoid constantly changing your hand position. Find the position that works best for you and stick with it.

The triceps extension belongs in the isolating exercise category because only the elbow joint is mobilized. As a result, the triceps extension does not recruit many muscles except the triceps and the forearm flexors. This exercise can be performed seated, standing, or lying on a bench, and with dumbbells, a barbell, or a pulley. You can work either one arm or both arms at a time.

How to Do It: Free Weights

While lying, seated, or standing, grab an EZ bar or a dumbbell with both hands (for bilateral work) or a dumbbell with one hand (for unilateral work). Lower the weight to your forehead (if lying) or behind your head (if seated or standing) with your elbows and pinkie fingers pointing toward the ceiling. Using your triceps, straighten your arms before bringing the weight back down. With dumbbells, you can shift from a neutral grip (thumbs facing down) in the stretched position to a pronated grip (thumbs facing each other) in the contracted position to better squeeze your triceps.

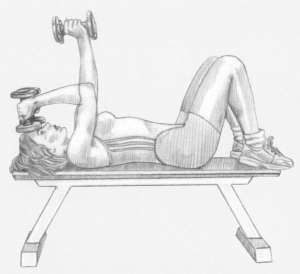

▌Lying triceps extension using dumbbells

How to Do It: Cable

You can use a high or low pulley to work either both arms at the same time or to alternate between arms. Attach a rope that you can grab with one or both hands. To work both arms at the same time, grab the rope and stand facing away from a high pulley with your feet staggered and your upper body leaning forward at about a 120-degree angle to the floor. Extend your arms straight ahead and then slowly bend them to lower the weight back down.

To work one arm at a time, stand perpendicular to a low pulley with your nonworking arm closer to the machine. Grab the rope behind your head with your elbow bent and extend your arm straight up; then slowly bend it to lower the weight back down.

❚ Start position

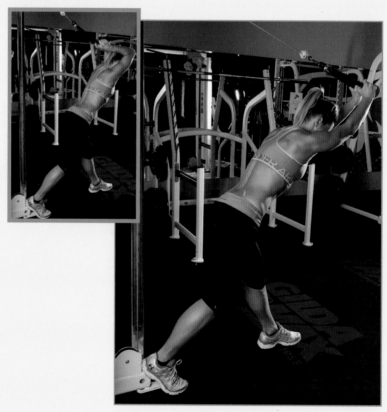

❚ Bilateral standing triceps extension at a high pulley

Start position

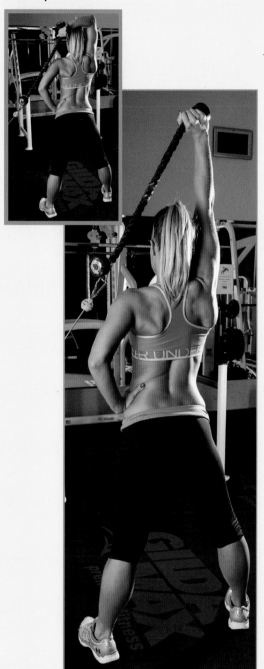

Triceps brachii
- Medial head
- Lateral head
- Long head

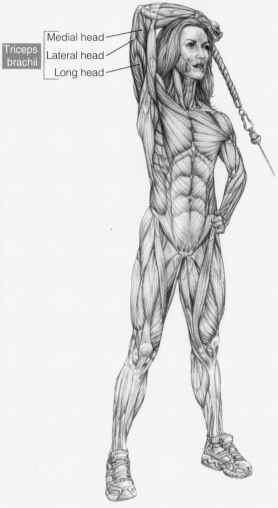

Unilateral standing triceps extension at a low pulley

Pro

- This exercise is unique in the category of triceps exercises in that it provides a good stretch.

Con

- With free weights, as fatigue sets in, it is easy to lose your form, arch your back, or hit yourself in the head with the weight.

- **With either dumbbells or a barbell, the elbow joints are heavily taxed during the extensions. You must really control the movement and perform it slowly to avoid hurting your elbow joint.**

- **If you feel any pain in your elbows as you extend your forearms, do not completely lock your arms because full extension may be damaging for some women. Instead, use continuous tension by stopping short of complete extension.**

Tips

- The farther your elbows are from your torso, the more you are going to recruit the long head of the triceps.

- Doing this exercise unilaterally creates a better stretch and a more pronounced contraction as a result of a greater range of motion.

- Performing this exercise standing forces you to arch your back, which may cause disc compressions. The seated position is safer. The lying position is the safest as far as back protection is concerned. Lying on a bench or on the floor not only protects your back but also improves your form by preventing you from swinging your torso.

FREE WEIGHTS OR MACHINE?

The pulley system makes machines safer for the elbows than free weights, but some triceps machines are tough on the joints anyway. If you suffer from any elbow joint pain, it is best to avoid this exercise or use only a complex cable machine.

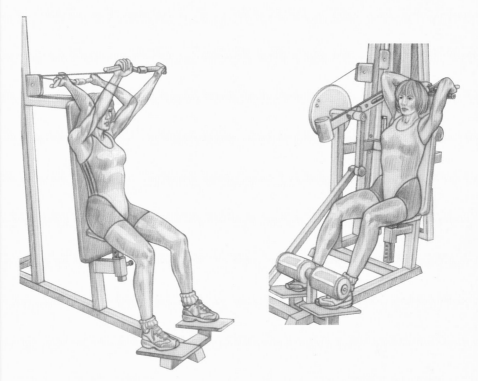

Two overhead triceps extension machine variations

TRICEPS KICKBACK

The triceps kickback belongs in the isolating exercise category because only the elbow joint is mobilized. As a result, the triceps kickback does not recruit many muscles except the triceps and the forearm flexors.

How to Do It

This exercise can be done unilaterally or bilaterally (this description is of the unilateral version). While leaning forward, grab a dumbbell with your hand in the neutral position (thumb pointing forward). In the starting position, your upper arm should be close to your side and roughly parallel to the floor. The elbow is bent to about a 90-degree angle with the upper arm. Using your triceps, straighten your arm along your side. Hold the position for at least one second with the arm extended before lowering the weight.

   The unilateral version places less stress on the lower back and allows you to perform the movement in a stricter manner with perfect technique. The bilateral version takes less time.

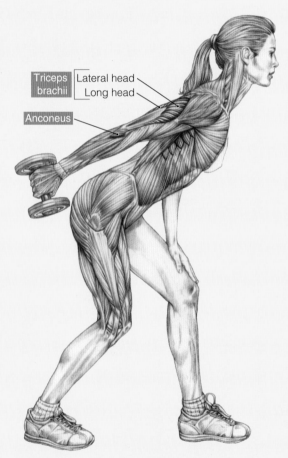

Triceps brachii — Lateral head
— Long head

Anconeus

❚ Unilateral triceps kickback using a dumbbell

Pro

- Of all the free-weight triceps exercises, this one is the safest on the elbow. You should be able to perform triceps kickbacks even if your elbows hurt a little when you do other triceps exercises.

Con

- Little muscle stretch is provided by this exercise, so some women have difficulty feeling the triceps contraction.

- **The lower back is pressured as a result of the bent-over position when you do this exercise bilaterally. However, if you perform the kickback one arm at a time, you can press your free hand against your thigh, which will help support your spine.**
- **As with any triceps exercise, if any pain occurs, stop and let your joints recover for several days before resuming triceps training!**

Tips

- Hold the extended position as long as possible to contract your triceps as much as possible. In fact, you have to generate a lot of muscle tension to keep your arms extended during this exercise—unlike with other triceps exercises. Take advantage of this!
- You can focus the work on the outside portion of your triceps by turning your pinkie finger slightly to the outside in the contracted position.

Cable Variation

Instead of dumbbells, you can use a low pulley. The main advantage of the pulley is that it provides more continuous and fluid tension than free weights do.

▌ **Start position**

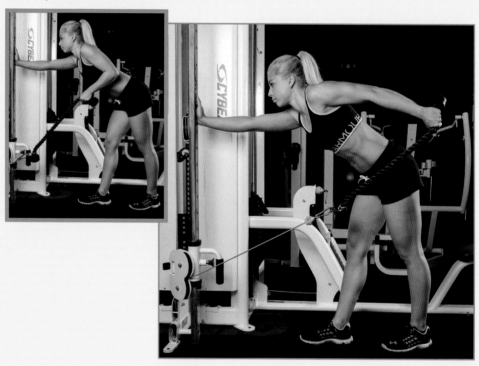

▌ **Unilateral triceps kickback at a low pulley**

- **Biceps:** Place one hand on the back of a chair and turn your back very slowly toward the chair. Rotate your wrist from left to right and then right to left to stretch the two heads of the biceps. Your biceps is in a very vulnerable position whenever it is stretched, so avoid any jerky movements.

- **Triceps:** Lift one arm so that your biceps is right next to your head. Pull on your elbow with the other hand so that your arm bends as much as possible. Ideally, the hand of your stretched arm would touch that side's shoulder while your elbow is placed as high as possible.

- **Forearms:** With your arms bent, put the palms of your hands together with your fingers pointing up so you can stretch the forearm flexors. With your arms bent, put the back of your hands together with your fingers pointing down so you can stretch the extensors.

- **Forearms:** Alternatively, you can stretch one forearm at a time by flexing or extending one hand with the other while keeping your arms relatively straight.

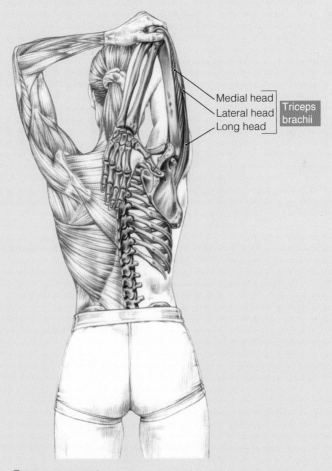

Medial head
Lateral head
Long head

Triceps brachii

Triceps stretch

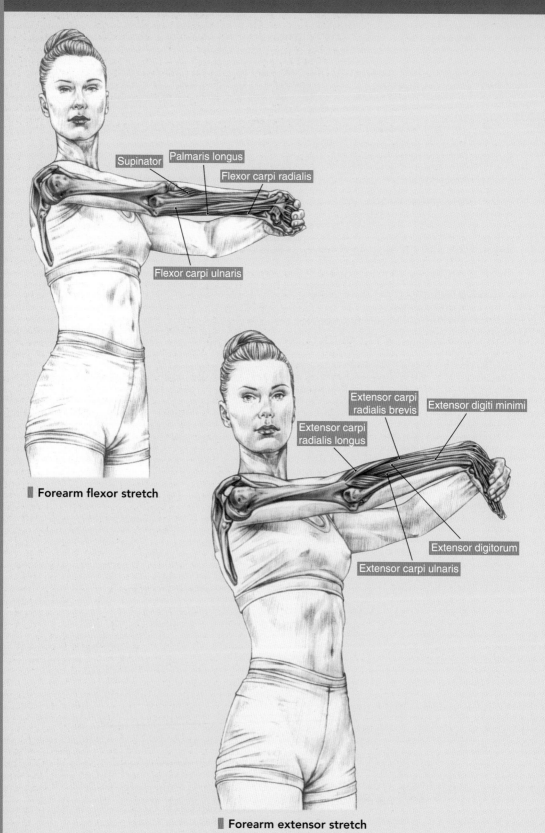

Supinator
Palmaris longus
Flexor carpi radialis
Flexor carpi ulnaris

▍ Forearm flexor stretch

Extensor carpi radialis brevis
Extensor digiti minimi
Extensor carpi radialis longus
Extensor digitorum
Extensor carpi ulnaris

▍ Forearm extensor stretch

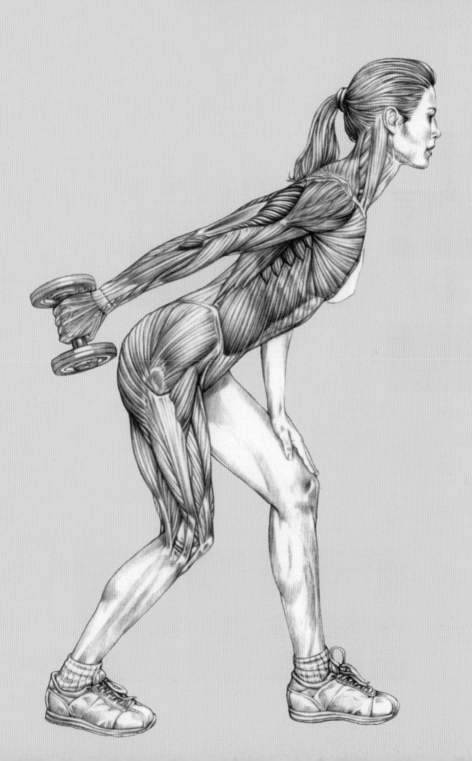

BEGINNER PROGRAMS

The goal of these programs is to wake up your muscles and joints and expose them to training. Avoid doing too much exercise too soon; otherwise you may experience long lasting and painful soreness. These programs are perfect if you have little time to train and no athletic background.

Minimal Equipment, Whole Body

LEGS
1. Lunge: 2 or 3 sets of 20 repetitions per leg, p. 99

BACK
2. Dumbbell row: 2 or 3 sets of 20 repetitions, p. 223

SHOULDERS
3. Bent-over dumbbell lateral raise: 2 or 3 sets of 20 repetitions, p. 211

ABDOMINALS
4. Crunch: 2 or 3 sets of 20 repetitions, p. 162

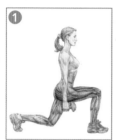 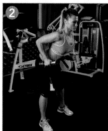 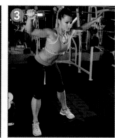 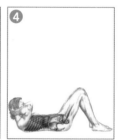

After a few weeks, move on to a more challenging program:

LEGS
1. Lunge: 3 or 4 sets of 20 repetitions per leg, p. 99
2. Stiff-leg dumbbell deadlift: 3 or 4 sets of 20 repetitions, p. 114

BACK
3. Dumbbell row: 3 or 4 sets of 20 repetitions, p. 223

SHOULDERS
4. Bent-over dumbbell lateral raise: 2 or 3 sets of 20 repetitions, p. 211

ABDOMINALS
5. Crunch: 3 or 4 sets of 20 repetitions, p. 162

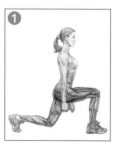 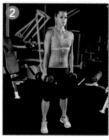 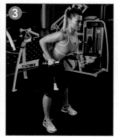 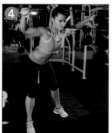 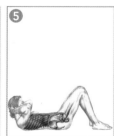

Gym Equipment, Whole Body

LEGS
① Barbell squat: 3 or 4 sets of 20 repetitions, p. 78

BACK
② Barbell row: 2 or 3 sets of 20 repetitions, p. 224

SHOULDERS
③ Cable lateral raise: 2 or 3 sets of 20 repetitions, p. 202

ABDOMINALS
④ Crunch: 2 or 3 sets of 20 repetitions, p. 162

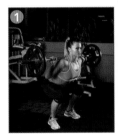 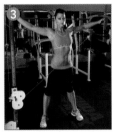 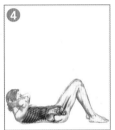 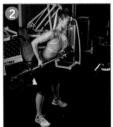

After a few weeks, move on to a more challenging program:

LEGS
① Barbell squat: 3 or 4 sets of 20 repetitions, p. 78
② Stiff-leg barbell deadlift: 3 or 4 sets of 20 repetitions, p. 114

BACK
③ Barbell row: 3 or 4 sets of 20 repetitions, p. 224

SHOULDERS
④ Cable lateral raise: 2 or 3 sets of 20 repetitions, p. 202

ABDOMINALS
⑤ Crunch: 3 or 4 sets of 20 repetitions, p. 162

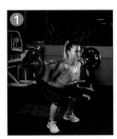 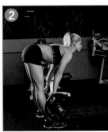 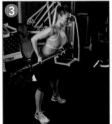 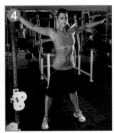 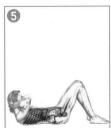

Machines Only, Whole Body

LEGS
1 Leg press: 3 or 4 sets of 20 repetitions, p. 96

BACK
2 Wide-grip cable pull-down: 2 or 3 sets of 20 repetitions, p. 228

SHOULDERS
3 Machine lateral raise: 2 or 3 sets of 20 repetitions, p. 200

ABDOMINALS
4 Machine crunch: 2 or 3 sets of 20 repetitions, p. 170

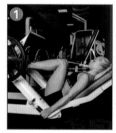 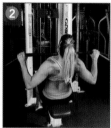 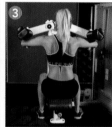 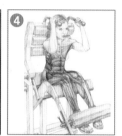

After a few weeks, move on to a more challenging program:

LEGS
1 Leg press: 3 or 4 sets of 20 repetitions, p. 96
2 Machine leg curl: 3 or 4 sets of 20 repetitions, p. 121

BACK
3 Wide-grip cable pull-down: 3 or 4 sets of 20 repetitions, p. 228

SHOULDERS
4 Machine lateral raise: 2 or 3 sets of 20 repetitions, p. 200

ABDOMINALS
5 Machine crunch: 3 or 4 sets of 20 repetitions, p. 170

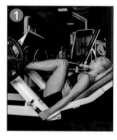 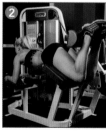 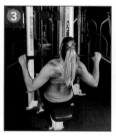 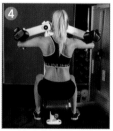 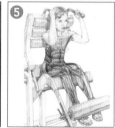

Minimal Equipment, Lower Body

LEGS

1. Dumbbell squat: 3 or 4 sets of 20 repetitions, p. 87
2. Lunge: 2 or 3 sets of 20 repetitions per leg, p. 99
3. Kneeling hip extension: 2 or 3 sets of 20 repetitions per leg, p. 45
4. Stiff-leg dumbbell deadlift: 3 or 4 sets of 20 repetitions, p.114

ABDOMINALS

5. Crunch: 3 or 4 sets of 20 repetitions, p. 162

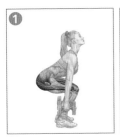 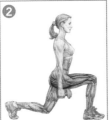 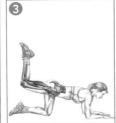 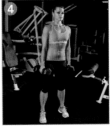 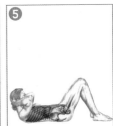

After a few weeks, move on to a more challenging program:

LEGS

1. Dumbbell squat: 2 or 3 sets of 20 repetitions, p. 87
2. Lunge: 2 or 3 sets of 20 repetitions per leg, p. 99
3. Kneeling hip extension: 2 or 3 sets of 20 repetitions per leg, p. 45

ABDOMINALS

4. Crunch: 3 or 4 sets of 20 repetitions, p. 162

LEGS

5. Stiff-leg dumbbell deadlift: 3 or 4 sets of 20 repetitions, p. 114
6. Bridge: 3 or 4 sets of 20 repetitions, p. 49

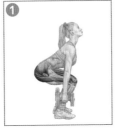 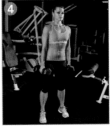 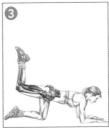 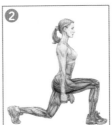 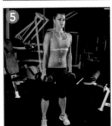 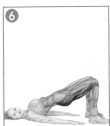

Gym Equipment, Lower Body

LEGS

1. Barbell squat: 2 or 3 sets of 20 repetitions, p. 78
2. One-leg butt press: 2 or 3 sets of 20 repetitions per leg, p. 53
3. Machine leg curl: 2 or 3 sets of 20 repetitions, p. 121

ABDOMINALS

4. Crunch: 2 or 3 sets of 20 repetitions, p. 162

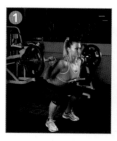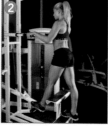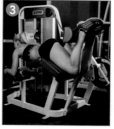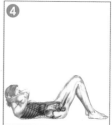

After a few weeks, move on to a more challenging program:

LEGS

1. Barbell squat: 3 or 4 sets of 20 repetitions, p. 78
2. Leg press: 3 or 4 sets of 20 repetitions, p. 96
3. One-leg butt press: 2 or 3 sets of 20 repetitions per leg, p. 53
4. Machine leg curl: 2 or 3 sets of 20 repetitions, p. 121

ABDOMINALS

5. Crunch: 3 or 4 sets of 20 repetitions, p. 162

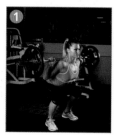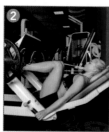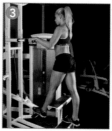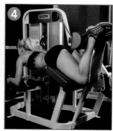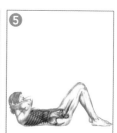

Minimal Equipment, Upper Body

BACK
1 Dumbbell row: 2 or 3 sets of 20 repetitions, p. 223

SHOULDERS
2 Bent-over dumbbell lateral raise: 2 or 3 sets of 20 repetitions, p. 211

CHEST
3 Incline dumbbell press: 2 or 3 sets of 20 repetitions, p. 261

ABDOMINALS
4 Crunch: 2 or 3 sets of 20 repetitions, p. 162

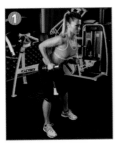 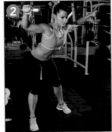 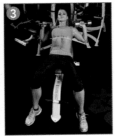 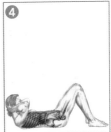

After a few weeks, move on to a more challenging program:

BACK
1 Dumbbell row: 2 or 3 sets of 20 repetitions, p. 223

SHOULDERS
2 Bent-over dumbbell lateral raise:
2 or 3 sets of
20 repetitions, p. 211

CHEST
3 Incline dumbbell press:
2 or 3 sets of
20 repetitions, p. 261

BICEPS
4 Dumbbell curl: 2 or 3 sets of 20 repetitions, p. 278

TRICEPS
5 Lying dumbbell triceps extension: 2 or 3 sets of
20 repetitions, p. 295

ABDOMINALS
6 Crunch: 3 or 4 sets of 20 repetitions, p. 162

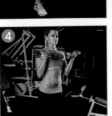 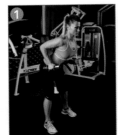 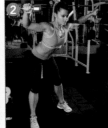 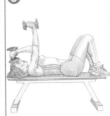 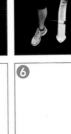 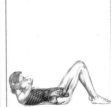

Gym Equipment, Upper Body

BACK
① Wide-grip cable pull-down: 2 or 3 sets of 20 repetitions, p. 228

SHOULDERS
② Machine lateral raise: 2 or 3 sets of 20 repetitions, p. 200

CHEST
③ Incline barbell press: 2 or 3 sets of 20 repetitions, p. 261

ABDOMINALS
④ Crunch: 2 or 3 sets of 20 repetitions, p. 162

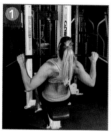
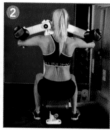
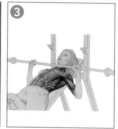
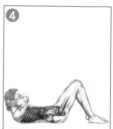

After a few weeks, move on to a more challenging program:

BACK
① Wide-grip cable pull-down: 2 or 3 sets of 20 repetitions, p. 228

SHOULDERS
② Machine lateral raise: 2 or 3 sets of 20 repetitions, p. 200

CHEST
③ Incline barbell press: 2 or 3 sets of 20 repetitions, p. 261

BICEPS
④ Dumbbell curl: 2 or 3 sets of 20 repetitions, p. 278

TRICEPS
⑤ Cable triceps extension: 2 or 3 sets of 20 repetitions, p. 296

ABDOMINALS
⑥ Crunch: 3 or 4 sets of 20 repetitions, p. 162

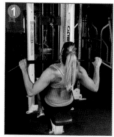
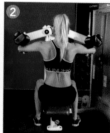
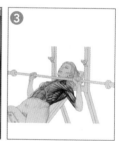
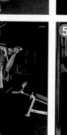
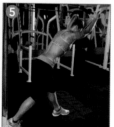
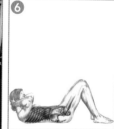

These programs are the place to start if you already have a little athletic background. The goal of these programs is to gently have your body acclimate to the strain weight training will induce.

Minimal Equipment, Whole Body: Lower Body and Upper Body on Separate Days

DAY 1: LOWER BODY

LEGS

1. Lunge: 2 or 3 sets of 20 repetitions per leg, p. 99
2. Stiff-leg dumbbell deadlift: 3 or 4 sets of 20 repetitions, p. 114
3. Kneeling hip extension: 2 or 3 sets of 20 repetitions per leg, p. 45

ABDOMINALS

4. Crunch: 2 or 3 sets of 20 repetitions, p. 162

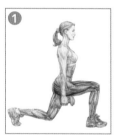 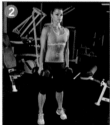 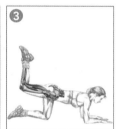 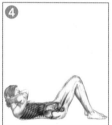

DAY 2: UPPER BODY

SHOULDERS

1. Bent-over dumbbell lateral raise: 2 or 3 sets of 20 repetitions, p. 211

BACK

2. Dumbbell row: 2 or 3 sets of 20 repetitions, p. 223

BICEPS

3. Dumbbell curl: 2 or 3 sets of 20 repetitions, p. 278

TRICEPS

4. Lying dumbbell triceps extension: 2 or 3 sets of 20 repetitions, p. 295

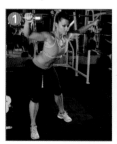 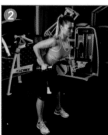 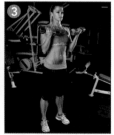 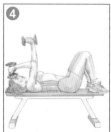

> continued

Minimal Equipment, Whole Body: Lower Body and Upper Body on Separate Days > continued

After a few weeks, move on to a more challenging program:

DAY 1: LOWER BODY

LEGS

1. Dumbbell squat: 2 or 3 sets of 20 repetitions, p. 87
2. Lunge: 2 or 3 sets of 20 repetitions per leg, p. 99
3. Stiff-leg dumbbell deadlift: 3 or 4 sets of 20 repetitions, p. 114
4. Kneeling hip extension: 2 or 3 sets of 20 repetitions per leg, p. 45

ABDOMINALS

5. Crunch: 2 or 3 sets of 20 repetitions, p. 162

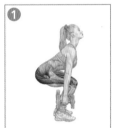
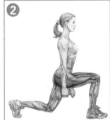
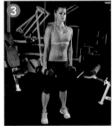
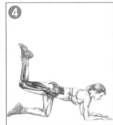
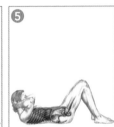

DAY 2: UPPER BODY

SHOULDERS

1. Bent-over dumbbell lateral raise: 3 or 4 sets of 20 repetitions, p. 211

BACK

2. Dumbbell row: 3 or 4 sets of 20 repetitions, p. 223

CHEST

3. Incline dumbbell press: 2 or 3 sets of 20 repetitions, p. 261

BICEPS

4. Dumbbell curl: 2 or 3 sets of 20 repetitions, p. 278

TRICEPS

5. Lying dumbbell triceps extension: 2 or 3 sets of 20 repetitions, p. 295

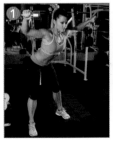
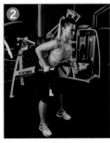
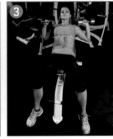
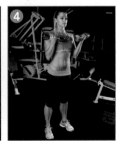
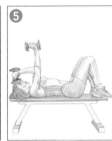

Minimal Equipment, Whole Body: Lower Body and Upper Body on Same Day

DAY 1: LOWER AND UPPER BODY

LOWER BODY

① Dumbbell squat: 2 or 3 sets of 20 repetitions, p. 87

② Kneeling hip extension: 2 or 3 sets of 20 repetitions per leg, p. 45

UPPER BODY

③ Crunch: 1 or 2 sets of 20 repetitions, p. 162

④ Bent-over dumbbell lateral raise: 2 or 3 sets of 20 repetitions, p. 211

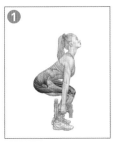 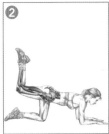 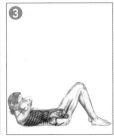 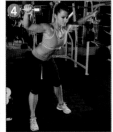

DAY 2: LOWER AND UPPER BODY

LOWER BODY

① Kneeling hip extension: 2 or 3 sets of 20 repetitions per leg, p. 45

② Stiff-leg dumbbell deadlift: 3 or 4 sets of 20 repetitions, p. 114

UPPER BODY

③ Crunch: 1 or 2 sets of 20 repetitions, p. 162

④ Dumbbell row: 2 or 3 sets of 20 repetitions, p. 223

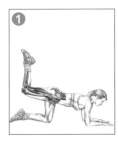 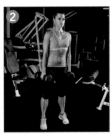 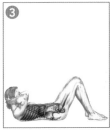 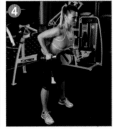

Gym Equipment, Whole Body: Lower Body and Upper Body on Separate Days

DAY 1: LOWER BODY

LEGS
1. Leg press: 2 or 3 sets of 20 repetitions, p. 96
2. One-leg butt press: 2 or 3 sets of 20 repetitions per leg, p. 53
3. Machine leg curl: 2 or 3 sets of 20 repetitions, p. 121

ABDOMINALS
4. Crunch: 2 or 3 sets of 20 repetitions, p. 162

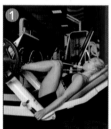 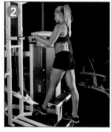 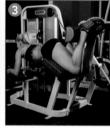 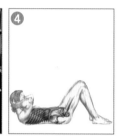

DAY 2: UPPER BODY

BACK
1. Wide-grip cable pull-down: 2 or 3 sets of 20 repetitions, p. 228

SHOULDERS
2. Machine lateral raise: 2 or 3 sets of 20 repetitions, p. 200

CHEST
3. Incline barbell press: 2 or 3 sets of 20 repetitions, p. 261

BICEPS
4. Low-pulley curl: 2 or 3 sets of 20 repetitions, p. 280

TRICEPS
5. Cable triceps extension: 2 or 3 sets of 20 repetitions, p. 296

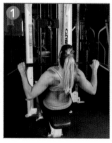 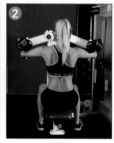 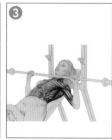 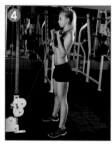 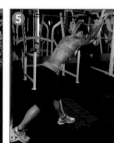

After a few weeks, move on to a more challenging program:

DAY 1: LOWER BODY

LEGS
1. Barbell squat: 3 or 4 sets of 20 repetitions, p. 78
2. Stiff-leg dumbbell deadlift: 3 or 4 sets of 20 repetitions, p. 114
3. Leg press: 2 or 3 sets of 20 repetitions, p. 96
4. Machine leg curl: 2 or 3 sets of 20 repetitions, p. 121

ABDOMINALS
5. Machine crunch: 2 or 3 sets of 20 repetitions, p. 170

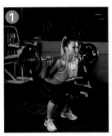 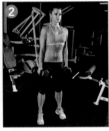 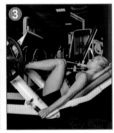 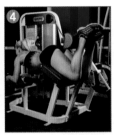 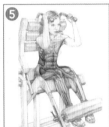

DAY 2: UPPER BODY

BACK
1. Wide-grip cable pull-down: 3 or 4 sets of 20 repetitions, p. 228

SHOULDERS
2. Machine lateral raise: 3 or 4 sets of 20 repetitions, p. 200

CHEST
3. Incline barbell press: 2 or 3 sets of 20 repetitions, p. 261

BICEPS
4. Low-pulley curl: 3 or 4 sets of 20 repetitions, p. 280

TRICEPS
5. Cable triceps extension: 3 or 4 sets of 20 repetitions, p. 296

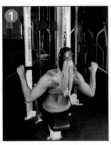 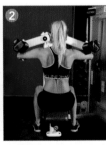 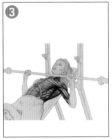 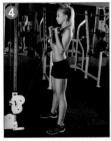 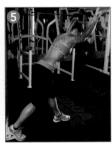

Gym Equipment, Whole Body: Lower Body and Upper Body on Same Day

DAY 1: LOWER BODY AND UPPER BODY

LOWER BODY

1. Leg press: 2 or 3 sets of 20 repetitions, p. 96
2. Machine hip extension: 2 or 3 sets of 20 repetitions per leg, p. 48

UPPER BODY

3. Machine crunch: 1 or 2 sets of 20 repetitions, p. 170
4. Machine lateral raise: 2 or 3 sets of 20 repetitions, p. 200

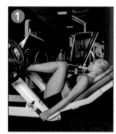 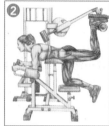 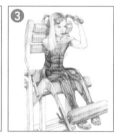 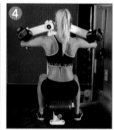

DAY 2: LOWER BODY AND UPPER BODY

LOWER BODY

1. One-leg butt press: 2 or 3 sets of 20 repetitions per leg, p. 53
2. Stiff-leg dumbbell deadlift: 3 or 4 sets of 20 repetitions, p. 114

UPPER BODY

3. Machine crunch: 1 or 2 sets of 20 repetitions, p. 170
4. Machine row: 2 or 3 sets of 20 repetitions, p. 227

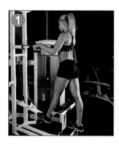 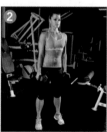 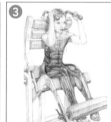 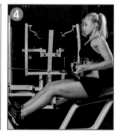

Minimal Equipment, Lower Body

DAY 1

LEGS

1. Dumbbell squat: 3 or 4 sets of 20 repetitions, p. 87
2. Kneeling hip extension: 2 or 3 sets of 20 repetitions per leg, p. 45
3. Stiff-leg dumbbell deadlift: 3 or 4 sets of 20 repetitions, p. 114

ABDOMINALS

4. Crunch: 3 or 4 sets of 20 repetitions, p.162

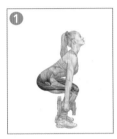 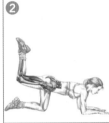 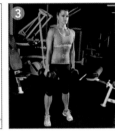 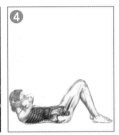

DAY 2

LEGS

1. Lunge: 2 or 3 sets of 20 repetitions per leg, p. 99
2. Bridge: 3 or 4 sets of 20 repetitions, p. 49
3. Stiff-leg dumbbell deadlift: 3 or 4 sets of 20 repetitions, p. 114

ABDOMINALS

4. Crunch: 3 or 4 sets of 20 repetitions, p.162

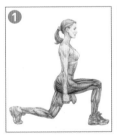 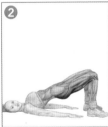 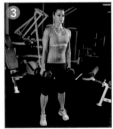 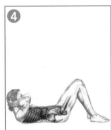

> continued

Minimal Equipment, Lower Body > continued

After a few weeks, move on to a more challenging program:

DAY 1

LEGS

1. Dumbbell squat: 3 or 4 sets of 20 to 15 repetitions, p. 87
2. Kneeling hip extension: 3 or 4 sets of 20 repetitions per leg, p. 45
3. Stiff-leg dumbbell deadlift: 3 or 4 sets of 20 to 15 repetitions, p. 114

ABDOMINALS

4. Crunch: 3 or 4 sets of 20 repetitions, p. 162

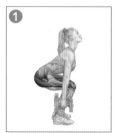 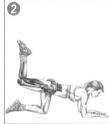 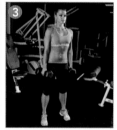 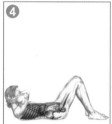

DAY 2

LEGS

1. Lunge: 3 or 4 sets of 20 repetitions per leg, p. 99
2. Bridge: 3 or 4 sets of 20 repetitions, p. 49
3. Stiff-leg dumbbell deadlift: 3 or 4 sets of 20 to 15 repetitions, p. 114

ABDOMINALS

4. Crunch: 3 or 4 sets of 20 repetitions, p. 162

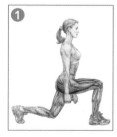 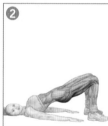 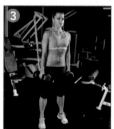 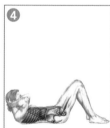

Gym Equipment, Lower Body

DAY 1

LEGS

1. Barbell squat: 2 or 3 sets of 20 repetitions, p. 78
2. One-leg butt press: 2 or 3 sets of 20 repetitions per leg, p. 53
3. Machine hip extension: 2 or 3 sets of 20 repetitions per leg, p. 48

ABDOMINALS

4. Machine crunch: 2 or 3 sets of 20 repetitions, p. 170

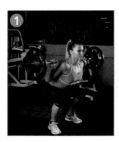
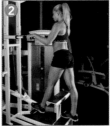
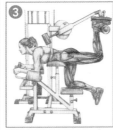
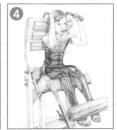

DAY 2

LEGS

1. Stiff-leg dumbbell deadlift: 2 or 3 sets of 20 repetitions, p. 114
2. Machine leg curl: 2 or 3 sets of 20 repetitions, p. 121
3. Leg press: 2 or 3 sets of 20 repetitions, p. 96

ABDOMINALS

4. Machine crunch: 2 or 3 sets of 20 repetitions, p. 170

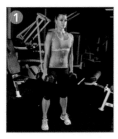
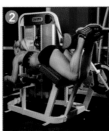
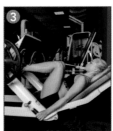
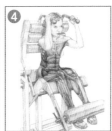

> continued

Gym Equipment, Lower Body > continued

After a few weeks, move on to a more challenging program:

DAY 1

LEGS

1. Barbell squat: 2 or 3 sets of 20 to 15 repetitions, p. 78
2. One-leg butt press: 2 or 3 sets of 20 repetitions per leg, p. 53
3. Machine hip extension: 2 or 3 sets of 20 repetitions per leg, p. 48
4. Leg press: 2 or 3 sets of 20 to 15 repetitions, p. 96

ABDOMINALS

5. Machine crunch: 2 or 3 sets of 20 repetitions, p. 170

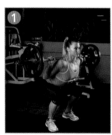 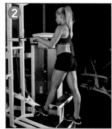 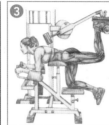 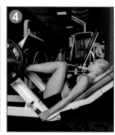 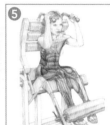

DAY 2

LEGS

1. Stiff-leg dumbbell deadlift: 2 or 3 sets of 20 repetitions, p. 114
2. One-leg butt press: 2 or 3 sets of 20 repetitions per leg, p. 53
3. Machine leg curl: 2 or 3 sets of 20 to 15 repetitions, p. 121
4. Leg press: 2 or 3 sets of 20 to 15 repetitions, p. 96

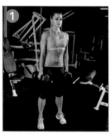 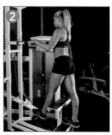 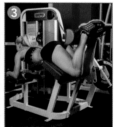 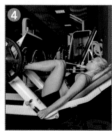

Minimal Equipment, Upper Body

DAY 1

BACK

1 Dumbbell row: 2 or 3 sets of 20 repetitions, p. 223

SHOULDERS

2 Bent-over dumbbell lateral raise: 2 or 3 sets of 20 repetitions, p. 211

TRICEPS

3 Lying dumbbell triceps extension: 2 or 3 sets of 20 repetitions, p. 295

ABDOMINALS

4 Crunch: 2 or 3 sets of 20 repetitions, p. 162

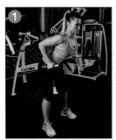 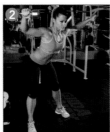 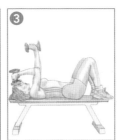 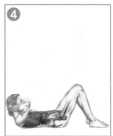

DAY 2

CHEST

1 Incline dumbbell press: 2 or 3 sets of 20 repetitions, p. 261

SHOULDERS

2 Dumbbell lateral raise: 2 or 3 sets of 20 repetitions, p. 196

3 Bent-over dumbbell lateral raise: 2 or 3 sets of 20 repetitions, p. 211

BICEPS

4 Dumbbell curl: 2 or 3 sets of 20 repetitions, p. 278

BACK

5 Dumbbell deadlift: 2 or 3 sets of 20 repetitions, p. 239

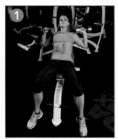 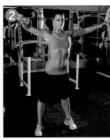 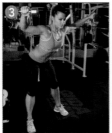 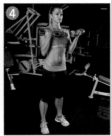 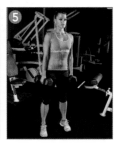

> continued

Minimal Equipment, Upper Body > continued

After a few weeks, move on to a more challenging program:

DAY 1

BACK
❶ Dumbbell row: 3 or 4 sets of 15 to 12 repetitions, p. 223

SHOULDERS
❷ Bent-over dumbbell lateral raise: 3 or 4 sets of 20 to 15 repetitions, p. 211

TRICEPS
❸ Lying dumbbell triceps extension: 3 or 4 sets of 20 to 15 repetitions, p. 295

ABDOMINALS
❹ Crunch: 2 or 3 sets of 20 repetitions, p. 162

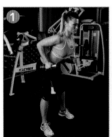 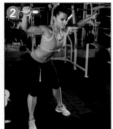 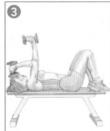 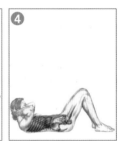

DAY 2

CHEST
❶ Incline dumbbell press: 2 or 3 sets of 15 to 12 repetitions, p. 261

SHOULDERS
❷ Bent-over dumbbell lateral raise: 3 or 4 sets of 20 to 15 repetitions, p. 212
❸ Dumbbell lateral raise: 2 or 3 sets of 20 to 15 repetitions, p. 196

BICEPS
❹ Dumbbell curl: 3 or 4 sets of 15 to 12 repetitions, p. 278

BACK
❺ Dumbbell deadlift: 2 or 3 sets of 20 to 15 repetitions, p. 239

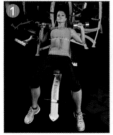 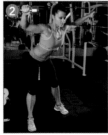 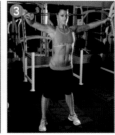 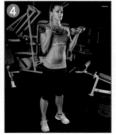 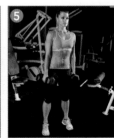

Gym Equipment, Upper Body

DAY 1

BACK

1. Wide-grip cable pull-down: 2 or 3 sets of 20 repetitions, p. 228

SHOULDERS

2. Machine lateral raise: 2 or 3 sets of 20 repetitions, p. 200
3. Bent-over cable lateral raise: 2 or 3 sets of 20 repetitions, p. 213

TRICEPS

4. Cable triceps extension: 2 or 3 sets of 20 repetitions, p. 296

ABDOMINALS

5. Machine crunch: 2 or 3 sets of 20 repetitions, p. 170

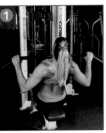 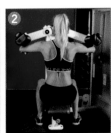 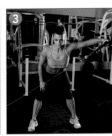 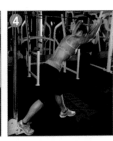 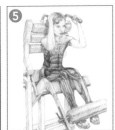

DAY 2

CHEST

1. Smith machine press: 2 or 3 sets of 20 repetitions, p. 259

SHOULDERS

2. Bent-over cable lateral raise: 3 or 4 sets of 20 repetitions, p. 213
3. Machine lateral raise: 2 or 3 sets of 20 repetitions, p. 200

BICEPS

4. Dumbbell curl: 2 or 3 sets of 20 repetitions, p. 278

LOWER BACK

5. Hyperextension: 2 or 3 sets of 20 repetitions, p. 245

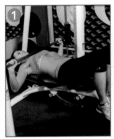 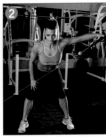 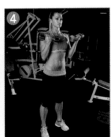 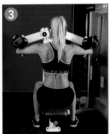 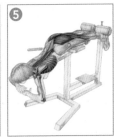

> continued

Gym Equipment, Upper Body > continued

After a few weeks, move on to a more challenging program:

DAY 1

BACK
1 Wide-grip cable pull-down: 3 or 4 sets of 15 to 12 repetitions, p. 228

SHOULDERS
2 Machine lateral raise: 3 or 4 sets of 20 to 15 repetitions, p. 200
3 Bent-over cable lateral raise: 2 or 3 sets of 20 to 15 repetitions, p. 213

TRICEPS
4 Cable triceps extension: 3 or 4 sets of 20 to 15 repetitions, p. 296

ABDOMINALS
5 Machine crunch: 2 or 3 sets of 20 repetitions, p. 170

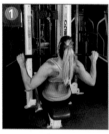 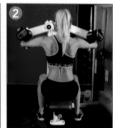 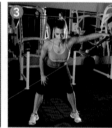 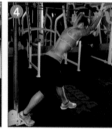 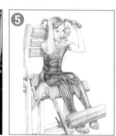

DAY 2

CHEST
1 Smith machine press: 3 or 4 sets of 15 to 12 repetitions, p. 259

SHOULDERS
2 Bent-over cable lateral raise: 3 or 4 sets of 20 to 15 repetitions, p. 213
3 Machine lateral raise: 2 or 3 sets of 20 to 15 repetitions, p. 200

BICEPS
4 Dumbbell curl: 3 or 4 sets of 15 to 12 repetitions, p. 278

LOWER BACK
5 Hyperextension: 2 or 3 sets of 20 repetitions, p. 245

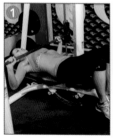 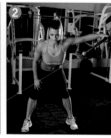 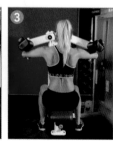 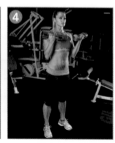 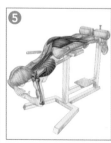

If you are not doing sport-specific training in addition to weight training, we recommend that you perform two weekly weight training workouts for a month or two, and then move to three sessions a week when you feel ready. At this point, your muscles should be used to your workouts and you should not suffer an excessive amount of soreness. You should also understand how to progressively increase the intensity of your workout (by lowering the number of repetitions to handle more weight) as well as the volume (by increasing the number of exercises or the number of sets per movement). These increases should be gradual to avoid overtraining.

Lower-Body Emphasis

DAY 1: LOWER BODY

LEGS
1. Leg press: 3 or 4 sets of 20-12 repetitions, p. 96
2. Stiff-leg dumbbell deadlift: 3 or 4 sets of 12 to 8 repetitions, p. 114
3. One-leg butt press: 2 or 3 sets of 20 repetitions per leg, p. 53
4. Machine leg curl: 3 or 4 sets of 15 to 12 repetitions, p. 121

ABDOMINALS
5. Machine crunch: 2 or 3 sets of 20 repetitions, p. 170

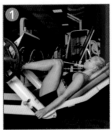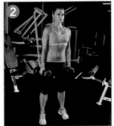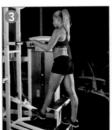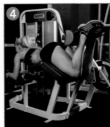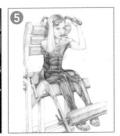

> continued

Lower-Body Emphasis > continued

DAY 2: UPPER BODY

BACK
① Wide-grip cable pull-down: 3 or 4 sets of 12 to 8 repetitions, p. 228

SHOULDERS
② Machine lateral raise: 3 or 4 sets of 15 to 12 repetitions, p. 200

CHEST
③ Incline barbell press: 3 or 4 sets of 12 to 8 repetitions, p. 261

BICEPS
④ Dumbbell curl: 3 or 4 sets of 15 to 12 repetitions, p. 278

TRICEPS
⑤ Cable triceps extension: 3 or 4 sets of 15 to 12 repetitions, p. 296

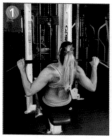 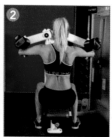 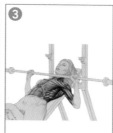 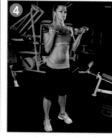 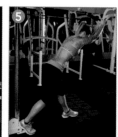

DAY 3: LOWER BODY

LEGS
① Barbell squat: 3 or 4 sets of 15 to 12 repetitions, p. 78
② Machine hip extension: 3 or 4 sets of 20 repetitions per leg, p. 48
③ Seated machine leg curl: 3 or 4 sets of 15 to 12 repetitions, p. 126

ABDOMINALS
④ Crunch: 3 or 4 sets of 20 repetitions, p. 162

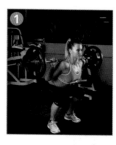 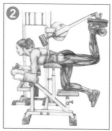 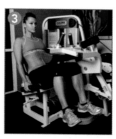 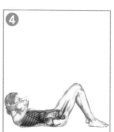

Upper-Body Emphasis

DAY 1: UPPER BODY

BACK

1. Wide-grip cable pull-down: 3 or 4 sets of 12 to 8 repetitions, p. 228

SHOULDERS

2. Machine lateral raise: 3 or 4 sets of 15 to 12 repetitions, p. 200

CHEST

3. Incline barbell press: 3 or 4 sets of 12 to 8 repetitions, p. 261

BICEPS

4. Dumbbell curl: 3 or 4 sets of 15 to 12 repetitions, p. 278

TRICEPS

5. Cable triceps extension: 3 or 4 sets of 15 to 12 repetitions, p. 296

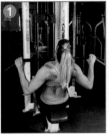 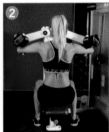 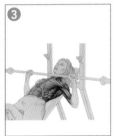 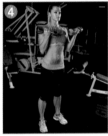 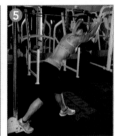

DAY 2: LOWER BODY

LEGS

1. Leg press: 3 or 4 sets of 20 to 12 repetitions, p. 96
2. One-leg butt press: 2 or 3 sets of 20 repetitions per leg, p. 53
3. Barbell squat: 3 or 4 sets of 15 to 12 repetitions, p. 78
4. Stiff-leg dumbbell deadlift: 3 or 4 sets of 12 to 8 repetitions, p. 114

ABDOMINALS

5. Machine crunch: 2 or 3 sets of 20 repetitions, p. 170

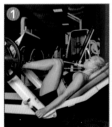 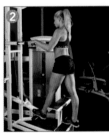 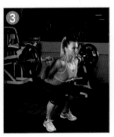 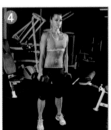 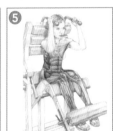

> continued

Upper-Body Emphasis > continued

DAY 3: UPPER BODY

SHOULDERS

1 Machine lateral raise: 3 or 4 sets of 12 to 8 repetitions, p. 200

CHEST

2 Incline barbell press: 3 or 4 sets of 12 to 8 repetitions, p. 261

BACK

3 Machine row: 3 or 4 sets of 12 to 8 repetitions, p. 227

TRICEPS

4 Cable triceps extension: 3 or 4 sets of 15 to 12 repetitions, p. 296

BICEPS

5 Dumbbell curl: 3 or 4 sets of 15 to 12 repetitions, p. 278

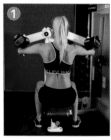 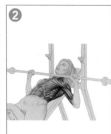 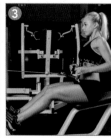 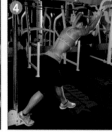 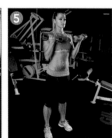

Whole-Body Emphasis

DAY 1: WHOLE BODY

LEGS

1. Barbell squat: 2 or 3 sets of 15 to 12 repetitions, p. 78
2. Leg press: 2 or 3 sets of 20 to 12 repetitions, p. 96

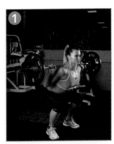
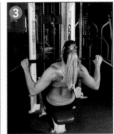
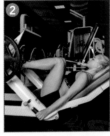

BACK

3. Wide-grip cable pull-down: 2 or 3 sets of 12 to 8 repetitions, p. 228

SHOULDERS

4. Machine lateral raise: 2 or 3 sets of 15 to 12 repetitions, p. 200

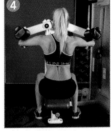
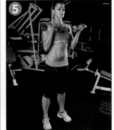
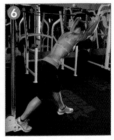

BICEPS

5. Dumbbell curl: 2 or 3 sets of 15 to 12 repetitions, p. 278

TRICEPS

6. Cable triceps extension: 2 or 3 sets of 15 to 12 repetitions, p. 296

DAY 2: WHOLE BODY

BACK

1. Machine row: 2 or 3 sets of 12 to 8 repetitions, p. 227

SHOULDERS

2. Machine lateral raise: 2 or 3 sets of 12 to 8 repetitions, p. 200

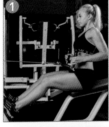
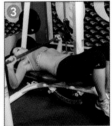
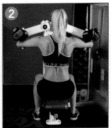

CHEST

3. Smith machine press: 2 or 3 sets of 12 to 8 repetitions, p. 259

LEGS

4. Leg press: 3 or 4 sets of 20 to 12 repetitions, p. 96

5. One-leg butt press: 2 or 3 sets of 20 repetitions per leg, p. 53

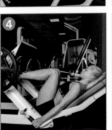
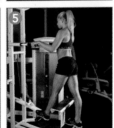
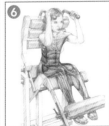

ABDOMINALS

6. Machine crunch: 2 or 3 sets of 20 repetitions, p. 170

> continued

Whole-Body Emphasis > continued

DAY 3: WHOLE BODY

LEGS

① Stiff-leg dumbbell deadlift: 3 or 4 sets of 12 to 8 repetitions, p. 114

② One-leg butt press: 2 or 3 sets of 20 repetitions per leg, p. 53

CHEST

③ Smith machine press: 3 or 4 sets of 12 to 8 repetitions, p. 259

BICEPS

④ Dumbbell curl: 2 or 3 sets of 15 to 12 repetitions, p. 278

TRICEPS

⑤ Cable triceps extension: 2 or 3 sets of 15 to 12 repetitions, p. 296

ABDOMINALS

⑥ Machine crunch: 2 or 3 sets of 20 repetitions, p. 170

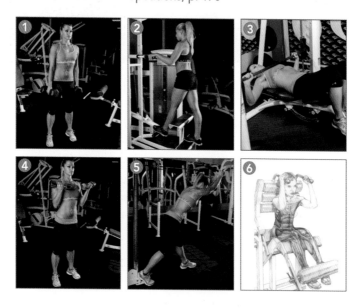

Lower Body Only

DAY 1

QUADRICEPS
1. Barbell squat: 3 or 4 sets of 15 to 12 repetitions, p. 78
2. Leg press: 3 or 4 sets of 20 to 12 repetitions, p. 96
3. Leg extension: 2 or 3 sets of 20 repetitions, p. 106

CALVES
4. Standing calf raise: 2 or 3 sets of 20 repetitions, p. 143

ABDOMINALS
5. Machine crunch: 2 or 3 sets of 20 repetitions, p. 170

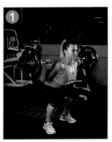 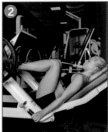 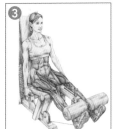 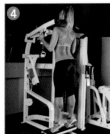 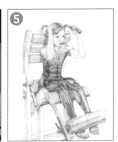

DAY 2

HAMSTRINGS
1. Stiff-leg dumbbell deadlift: 3 or 4 sets of 12 to 8 repetitions, p. 114
2. Prone machine leg curl: 2 or 3 sets of 15 to 12 repetitions, p. 121
3. Seated machine leg curl: 2 or 3 sets of 15 to 12 repetitions, p. 126

GLUTES
4. One-leg butt press: 3 or 4 sets of 20 repetitions per leg, p. 53

ABDOMINALS
5. Machine crunch: 2 or 3 sets of 20 repetitions, p. 170

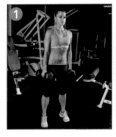 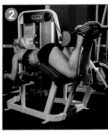 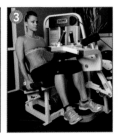 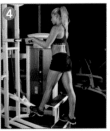 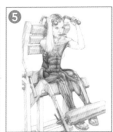

> continued

Lower Body Only > continued

DAY 3

GLUTES
① Machine leg extension: 3 or 4 sets of 20 repetitions per leg, p. 48
② One-leg butt press: 3 or 4 sets of 20 repetitions per leg, p. 53

QUADRICEPS
③ Barbell squat: 2 or 3 sets of 20 to 15 repetitions, p. 78
④ Leg press: 2 or 3 sets of 20 to 12 repetitions, p. 96

ABDOMINALS
⑤ Crunch: 3 or 4 sets of 20 repetitions, p. 162

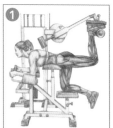 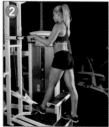 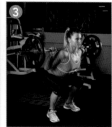 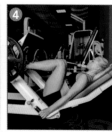 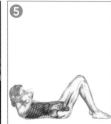

Upper Body Only

DAY 1

SHOULDERS

1. Machine lateral raise: 3 or 4 sets of 12 to 8 repetitions, p. 200
2. Bent-over dumbbell lateral raise: 3 or 4 sets of 12 to 8 repetitions, p. 211

CHEST

3. Incline dumbbell press: 4 or 5 sets of 12 to 8 repetitions, p. 261

ABDOMINALS

4. Crunch: 3 or 4 sets of 20 repetitions, p. 162

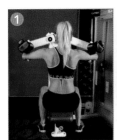
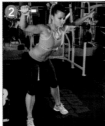
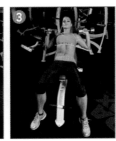
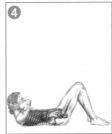

DAY 2

BACK

1. Machine row: 4 or 5 sets of 12 to 8 repetitions, p. 227

TRICEPS

2. Cable triceps extension: 3 or 4 sets of 15 to 12 repetitions, p. 296

BICEPS

3. Dumbbell curl: 3 or 4 sets of 15 to 12 repetitions, p. 278

ABDOMINALS

4. Crunch: 3 or 4 sets of 20 repetitions, p. 162

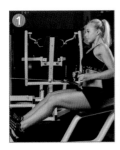
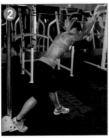
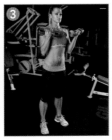
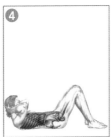

> continued

Upper Body Only > continued

DAY 3

SHOULDERS

1 Machine lateral raise: 3 or 4 sets of 12 to 8 repetitions, p. 200

CHEST

2 Incline dumbbell press: 4 or 5 sets of 12 to 8 repetitions, p. 261

BACK

3 Machine row: 4 or 5 sets of 12 to 8 repetitions, p. 227

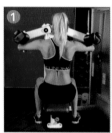 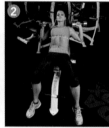 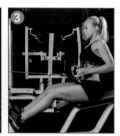

When you reach a point where your workouts are too cumbersome because you have to either perform too many sets or too many exercises to keep progressing, it may be time to add one more session per week. This increase will allow you to concentrate more on each body region because fewer muscles have to be trained during each workout.

Lower-Body Emphasis

DAY 1: LOWER BODY

LEGS

1. Leg press: 5 or 6 sets of 15 to10 repetitions, p. 96
2. Stiff-leg dumbbell deadlift: 4 or 5 sets of 12 to 8 repetitions, p. 114
3. One-leg butt press: 5 or 6 sets of 20 repetitions per leg, p. 53

ABDOMINALS

4. Machine crunch: 3 or 4 sets of 20 repetitions, p. 170

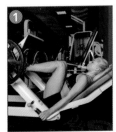 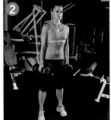 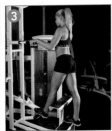 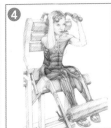

DAY 2: UPPER BODY

BACK

1. Wide-grip cable pull-down: 5 or 6 sets of 12 to 8 repetitions, p. 228

SHOULDERS

2. Machine lateral raise: 4 or 5 sets of 15 to 12 repetitions, p. 200

CHEST

3. Incline barbell press: 4 or 5 sets of 12-8 repetitions, p. 261

ABDOMINALS

4. Crunch: 3 or 4 sets of 20 repetitions, p. 162

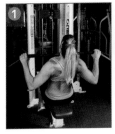 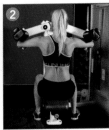 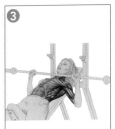 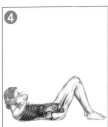

> continued

Lower-Body Emphasis > continued

DAY 3: LOWER BODY

LEGS

1. Barbell squat: 5 or 6 sets of 15 to 10 repetitions, p. 78
2. Machine leg extension: 5 or 6 sets of 20 repetitions per leg, p. 48
3. Seated machine leg curl: 3 or 4 sets of 15-12 repetitions, p. 126

ABDOMINALS

4. Lying leg raise: 2 or 3 sets of 20 repetitions, p. 172

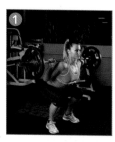 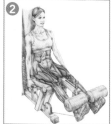 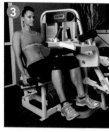 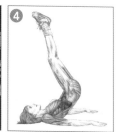

DAY 4: REAR LOWER BODY AND ARMS

LEGS

1. One-leg butt press: 5 or 6 sets of 20 repetitions per leg, p. 53
2. Prone machine leg curl: 5 or 6 sets of 15 to 12 repetitions, p.121
3. Bridge: 2 sets of 50 to 100 repetitions, p. 49

BICEPS

4. Dumbbell curl: 4 or 5 sets of 15 to 12 repetitions, p. 278

TRICEPS

5. Cable triceps extension: 5 or 6 sets of 15 to 12 repetitions, p. 296

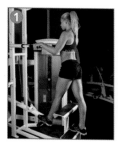 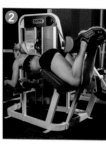 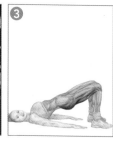 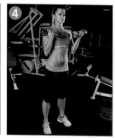 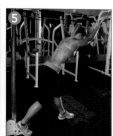

Upper-Body Emphasis

DAY 1: UPPER BODY

BACK
1. Wide-grip cable pull-down: 4 or 5 sets of 12 to 8 repetitions, p. 228

SHOULDERS
2. Machine lateral raise: 5 or 6 sets of 15 to 12 repetitions, p. 200

CHEST
3. Incline barbell press: 4 or 5 sets of 12 to 8 repetitions, p. 261

ABDOMINALS
4. Machine crunch: 2 or 3 sets of 20 repetitions, p. 170

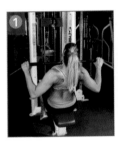 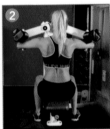 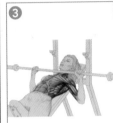 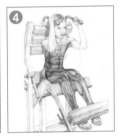

DAY 2: LOWER BODY

LEGS:
1. Leg press: 5 or 6 sets of 20 to 12 repetitions, p. 96
2. One-leg butt press: 4 or 5 sets of 20 repetitions per leg, p. 53
3. Barbell squat: 5 or 6 sets of 15 to 12 repetitions, p. 78

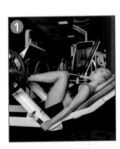 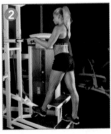 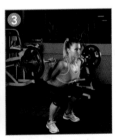

> continued

Upper-Body Emphasis > continued

DAY 3: UPPER BODY

SHOULDERS

① Machine lateral raise: 5 or 6 sets of 12 to 8 repetitions, p. 200

BICEPS

② Dumbbell curl: 4 or 5 sets of 15 to 12 repetitions, p. 278

TRICEPS

③ Cable triceps extension: 5 or 6 sets of 15 to 12 repetitions, p. 296

ABDOMINALS

④ Lying leg raise: 2 or 3 sets of 20 repetitions, p. 172

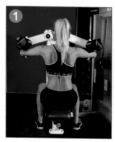 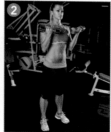 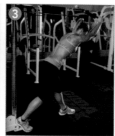 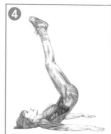

DAY 4: UPPER BODY

CHEST

① Incline barbell press: 5 or 6 sets of 12 to 8 repetitions, p. 261

BACK

② Machine row: 5 or 6 sets of 12 to 8 repetitions, p. 227

TRICEPS

③ Triceps kickback: 5 or 6 sets of 15 to 12 repetitions per arm, p. 300

BICEPS

④ Barbell curl: 3 or 4 sets of 15 to 12 repetitions, p. 280

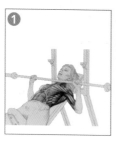 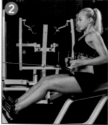 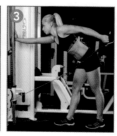 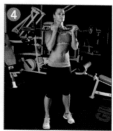

If you have little time to train or if you wish to tone up your body while getting rid of as much fat as possible, or both, circuits are the most appropriate form of training. Start with one session per week; as you progress, add more training days, performing the same circuit. You will know it is time to add more training days by closely monitoring your muscle strength. At first, if you do not have any athletic background, your muscles will feel tired for days after a workout. As you progress, their recovery will get faster and faster. When you do not need as much rest as before, it is time to add new training sessions.

Minimal Equipment, Whole Body

Do 1 or 2 circuits per workout without any rest between exercises. You should do 20 to 30 repetitions per set depending on your level of fitness.

1. Quadriceps: Lunge with the right and then with the left leg, p. 99
2. Upper back: Dumbbell row, p. 223
3. Shoulders: Bent-over dumbbell lateral raise, p. 211
4. Abdominals: Crunch, p. 162

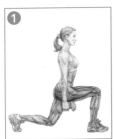
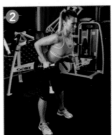
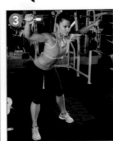
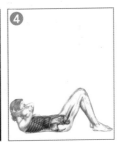

After a few weeks, move on to a more challenging circuit. Do 2 or 3 circuits per workout without any rest between exercises. You should do 20 to 30 repetitions per set.

1. Quadriceps: Lunge with the right and then with the left leg, p. 99
2. Hamstrings: Stiff-leg dumbbell deadlift, p. 114
3. Upper back: Dumbbell row, p. 223
4. Shoulders: Bent-over dumbbell lateral raise, p. 211
5. Abdominals: Crunch, p. 162

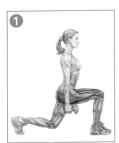
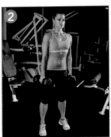
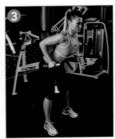
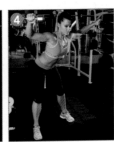
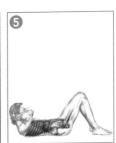

Gym Equipment, Whole Body

Do 1 or 2 circuits per workout without any rest between exercises. You should do 20 to 30 repetitions per set depending on your level of fitness.

1. Quadriceps: Barbell squat, p. 78
2. Upper back: Dumbbell row, p. 223
3. Shoulders: Machine lateral raise, p. 200
4. Abdominals: Machine crunch, p. 170

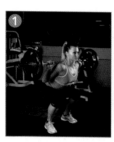 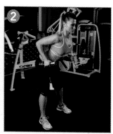 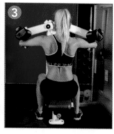 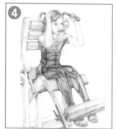

After a few weeks, move on to a more challenging circuit. Do 2 or 3 circuits per workout without any rest between exercises. You should do 20 to 30 repetitions per set.

1. Quadriceps: Barbell squat, p. 78
2. Hamstrings: Stiff-leg dumbbell deadlift, p. 114
3. Upper back: Dumbbell row, p. 223
4. Shoulders: Machine lateral raise, p. 200
5. Abdominals: Machine crunch, p. 170

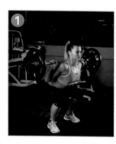 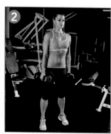 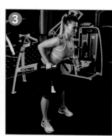 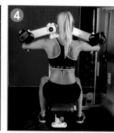 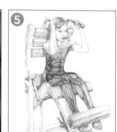

Minimal Equipment, Lower-Body Emphasis

Do 1 or 2 circuits per workout without any rest between exercises. You should do 20 to 30 repetitions per set depending on your level of fitness.

1. Quadriceps: Dumbbell squat, p. 87
2. Quadriceps: Lunge with the right and then with the left leg, p. 99
3. Glutes: Kneeling hip extension with the right and then with the left leg, p. 45
4. Hamstrings: Stiff-leg dumbbell deadlift, p. 114
5. Abdominals: Crunch, p. 162

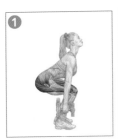 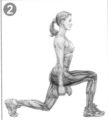 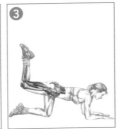 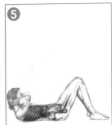 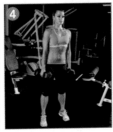

After a few weeks, move on to a more challenging circuit. Do 2 or 3 circuits per workout without any rest between exercises. You should do 20 to 30 repetitions per set.

1. Quadriceps: Dumbbell squat, p. 87
2. Quadriceps: Lunge with the right and then with the left leg, p. 99
3. Glutes: Kneeling hip extension with the right and then with the left leg, p. 45
4. Abdominals: Crunch, p. 162
5. Glutes: Bridge, p. 49
6. Hamstrings: Stiff-leg dumbbell deadlift, p. 114
7. Abdominals: Crunch, p. 162

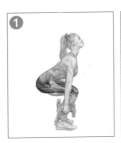 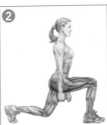 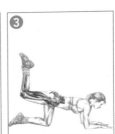

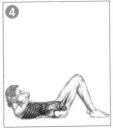 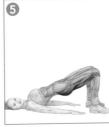 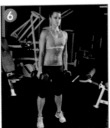 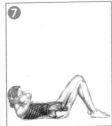

CIRCUIT TRAINING

Gym Equipment, Lower-Body Emphasis

Do 1 or 2 circuits per workout without any rest between exercises. You should do 20 to 30 repetitions per set depending on your level of fitness.

1 Quadriceps: Barbell squat, p. 78

2 Glutes: One-leg butt press with the right and then with the left leg, p. 53

3 Hamstrings: Machine leg curl, p. 121

4 Abdominals: Machine crunch, p. 170

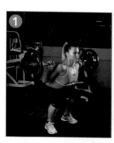 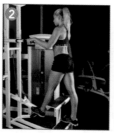 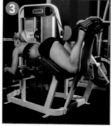 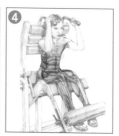

After a few weeks, move on to a more challenging circuit. Do 2 or 3 circuits per workout without any rest between exercises. You should do 20 to 30 repetitions per set.

1 Quadriceps: Barbell squat, p. 78

2 Quadriceps: Leg press, p. 96

3 Glutes: One-leg butt press with the right and then with the left leg, p. 53

4 Hamstrings: Machine leg curl, p. 121

5 Abdominals: Machine crunch, p. 170

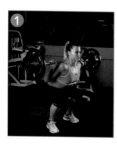 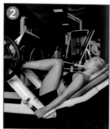 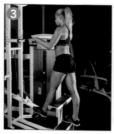 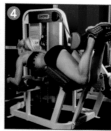 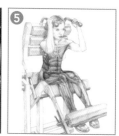

Minimal Equipment, Upper-Body Emphasis

Do 1 or 2 circuits per workout without any rest between exercises. You should do 10 to 20 repetitions per set depending on your level of fitness.

1. Shoulders: Bent-over dumbbell lateral raise, p. 211
2. Chest: Dumbbell press, p. 258
3. Back: Dumbbell row, p. 223
4. Abdominals: Crunch: p. 162

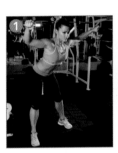
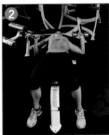
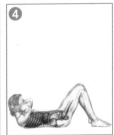

After a few weeks, move on to a more challenging circuit. Do 2 or 3 circuits per workout without any rest between exercises. You should do 15 to 20 repetitions per set.

1. Shoulders: Dumbbell lateral raise, p. 196
2. Chest: Dumbbell press, p. 258
3. Back: Dumbbell row, p. 223
4. Abdominals: Crunch, p. 162
5. Shoulders: Bent-over dumbbell lateral raise, p. 211
6. Biceps: Dumbbell curl, p. 278

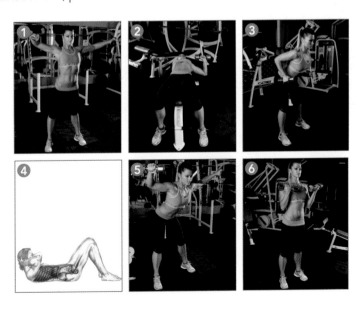
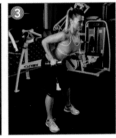

CIRCUIT TRAINING

Gym Equipment, Upper-Body Emphasis

Do 1 or 2 circuits per workout without any rest between exercises. You should do 10 to 20 repetitions per set depending on your level of fitness.

1. Shoulders: Machine lateral raise, p. 200
2. Chest: Smith machine press, p. 259
3. Back: Machine row, p. 227
4. Abdominals: Crunch, p. 162

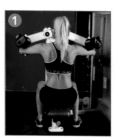
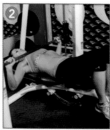
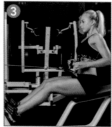
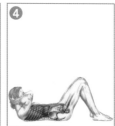

After a few weeks, move on to a more challenging circuit. Do 2 or 3 circuits per workout without any rest between exercises. You should do 15 to 20 repetitions per set.

1. Shoulders: Machine lateral raise, p. 200
2. Chest: Smith machine press, p. 259
3. Back: Machine row, p. 227
4. Abdominals: Crunch, p. 162
5. Shoulders: Bent-over cable lateral raise, p. 213
6. Biceps: Machine curl, p. 283

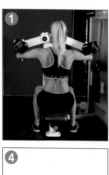
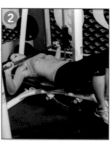
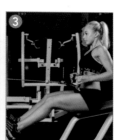
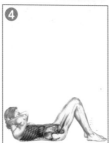
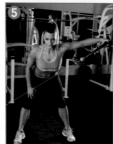
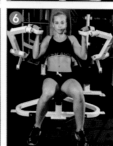

Specialized Home Circuits

If you do not want to spend too much time in the gym or if you do not have time to go to the gym on a particular day, here are two circuits you can perform at home once or twice a week. You can also add these circuits to your regular program on the off days in order to burn more fat while targeting the main problem areas in many women: the belly and the glutes.

HOME CIRCUIT FOR A FLAT ABDOMEN

This program is for flattening the abdominal muscles, losing belly fat, and slimming down the waist. Because no equipment is required, you can do it at home in the morning so that blood is circulating in your abdominal muscles throughout the day. Another option is to do it at home in the evening. Do 2 to 4 circuits per workout without any rest between exercises. Your repetitions will be a little more dynamic than normal, but you should still avoid any jerky movements, particularly of the lower back. You should do 25 to 50 repetitions per set depending on your level of fitness.

BEGINNER CIRCUIT

1 Crunch, p. 162
2 Oblique crunch, p. 168

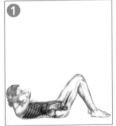
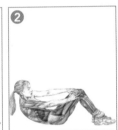

ADVANCED CIRCUIT

1 Lying leg raise, p. 172
2 Crunch, p. 162
3 Oblique crunch, p. 168

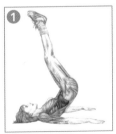
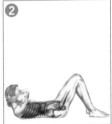
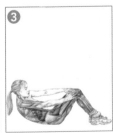

HOME CIRCUIT FOR SHAPING THE BUTTOCKS

This program is for shaping and rounding the buttocks. Because no equipment is required, you can do it at home in the morning so that blood is circulating in your glute muscles throughout the day. Another option is to do it at home in the evening. Do 2 to 4 circuits per workout without any rest between exercises. You should do 25 to 50 repetitions per set depending on your level of fitness.

BEGINNER CIRCUIT

1. Kneeling hip extension with one leg and then the other, p. 45
2. Bridge, p. 49

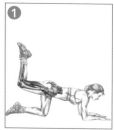 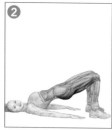

ADVANCED CIRCUIT

1. Lunge with one leg and then the other, p. 99
2. Kneeling hip extension with one leg and then the other, p. 45
3. Bridge, p. 49

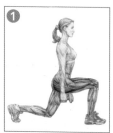 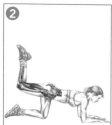 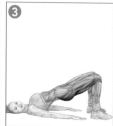

References

Introduction

1. Rønnestad, B.R. and I. Mujika. 2013. Optimizing strength training for running and cycling endurance performance: A review. *Scandinavian Journal of Medicine & Science in Sports.*

2. Jidovtseff, B. et al. 2013. The use of resistance training in amateur level team sports: The example of female handball. *Science & Sports* 28 (5): 281.

3. Perls, T. and D. Terry. 2003. Understanding the determinants of exceptional longevity. *Annals of Internal Medicine* 139(5, Pt 2):445-449.

4. Veerman, J.L., et al. 2012. Television viewing time and reduced life expectancy: A life table analysis. *British Journal of Sports Medicine.* 46 (13):927-930.

5. Wen, C.P. et al. 2011. Minimum amount of physical activity for reduced mortality and extended life expectancy: A prospective cohort study. *The Lancet* 378 (9798): 1244-1253.

Developing Your Own Training Program

1. Miller, B.F. et al. 2007. Tendon collagen synthesis at rest and after exercise in women. *Journal of Applied Physiology* 102 (2): 541-546.

2. Westcott, W.L. et al. 2001. Effects of regular and slow speed resistance training on muscle strength. *Journal of Sports Medicine and Physical Fitness* 41 (2): 154-158.

3. Kenneth, J. et al. 2013. Effect of brief daily resistance training on rapid force development in painful neck and shoulder muscles: Randomized controlled trial. *Clinical Physiology and Functional Imaging* 33 (5): 386-392.

4. Applegate, M. 2013. Gender differences in training volumes, blood lactate, and perceptual responses during the free weight bench press performed utilizing variable loads and recovery durations. *Journal of Strength and Conditioning Research* 27 (Suppl. 4): S91.

5. Medema-Johnson, H. 2013. The effect of self-paced and assigned between-set recovery durations on performance of the free weight bench press in trained lifters. *Journal of Strength and Conditioning Research* 27 (Suppl. 4): S91.

6. Smith, A. 2006. Comparison of free weights and machine weights for enhancing bench press strength in young women. *Journal of Strength and Conditioning Research* 20 (4): e32.

7. Pujol, T.J. 2012. Effect of free-weight and machine-weight training on upper-body strength gains in low- and high-strength college women. *Medicine & Science in Sports & Exercise* 44 (5S): 606.

8. Hill, J.L. 2013. Effect of free-weight and machine-weight training on upper-body strength gains in low-fat and high-fat college women. *Medicine & Science in Sports & Exercise* 45 (5S): 592.

9. Smith, M.M., A.J Sommer, B.E. Starkoff, and S.T. Devor. 2013. Crossfit-based high-intensity power training improves maximal aerobic fitness and body composition. *Journal of Strength & Conditioning Research* 27 (11): 3159-3172.

10. Burrows, N.J. 2013. The effect of a single bout of resistance exercise on pain sensitivity in knee osteoarthritis. *Medicine & Science in Sports & Exercise* 45 (5S): 647.

11. Giuseppe, F. 2013. Analysis of results at 5-year follow-up in a large cohort of patients treated with matrix-assisted autologous chondrocyte transplantation. Does patient sex influence cartilage surgery outcome? *American Journal of Sports Medicine* 41 (8): 1827-1834.

12. Willis, L.H. 2102. Effects of aerobic and/or resistance training on body mass and fat mass in overweight or obese adults. *Journal of Applied Physiology* 113 (12): 1831-1837.

13. Tan, J. 2013. Effects of a single bout of lower body aerobic exercise on muscle activation and performance during subsequent lower- and upper-body resistance exercise workouts. *Journal of Strength and Conditioning Research* 27 (Suppl. 4): S22.

14. Shostak, A. et al. 2013. Circadian regulation of lipid mobilization in white adipose tissues. *Diabetes* 62 (7): 2195-2203.

15. Haxhi, J. 2013. Is timing important? *Annals of Nutrition and Metabolism* 62: 14-25.

16. Holmstrup, M.E., et al. 2014. Multiple short bouts of exercise over 12-h period reduce glucose excursions more than an energy-matched single bout of exercise. *Metabolism—Clinical and Experimental* 63 (4): 510-519.

REFERENCES

17. Church, T.S. et al. 2009. Changes in weight, waist circumference and compensatory responses with different doses of exercise among sedentary, overweight postmenopausal women. *PLOS ONE* 4 (2): e4515.
18. Melanson, E.L. 2013. Resistance to exercise-induced weight loss: Compensatory behavioral adaptations. *Medicine & Science in Sports & Exercise* 45 (8): 1600-1609.
19. Blonc, S. et al. 2010. Effects of 5 weeks of training at the same time of day on the diurnal variations of maximal muscle power performance. *Journal of Strength and Conditioning Research* 24 (1): 23-29.
20. Rønnestad, B.R. et al. 2011. Effects of in-season strength maintenance training frequency in professional soccer players. *Journal of Strength and Conditioning Research* 25 (10): 2653-60.
21. Cramer, J.T. et al. 2004. Acute effects of static stretching on peak torque in women. *Journal of Strength and Conditioning Research* 18 (2): 236-241.
22. Chenevière, X. et al. 2010. Differences in whole-body fat oxidation kinetics between cycling and running. *European Journal of Applied Physiology* 109 (6):1037-45.

Round Your Glutes

1. Bartlett, J.L. 2014. Activity and functions of the human gluteal muscles in walking, running, sprinting, and climbing. *American Journal of Physical Anthropology* 153 (1): 124-131.
2. Stallknecht, B. 2007. Are blood flow and lipolysis in subcutaneous adipose tissue influenced by contractions in adjacent muscles in humans? *American Journal of Physiology—Endocrinology and Metabolism* 292 (2): E394-399.
3. Heinonen, I. 2012. Regulation of subcutaneous adipose tissue blood flow during exercise in humans. *Journal of Applied Physiology* 112: 1059-1063.
4. Lee, J.H. et al. 2014. Different hip rotations influence hip abductor muscles activity during isometric side-lying hip abduction in subjects with gluteus medius weakness. *Journal of Electromyography & Kinesiology* 24 (2): 318-324.
5. Hafiz, E. 2013. Do anatomical or other hip characteristics predispose to lower limb musculoskeletal injury? A systematic review. *Medicine & Science in Sports & Exercise* 45 (Suppl. 1) 5S: 5.

Trim Your Calves

1. Bird, M.L. et al. 2012. Serum [25(OH)D] status, ankle strength and activity show seasonal variation in older adults: Relevance for winter falls in higher latitudes. *Age and Ageing* 42 (2): 181-185.

Flatten Your Abs

1. Mole, J.L. et al. 2014. The effect of transversus abdominis activation on exercise-related transient abdominal pain. *Journal of Science and Medicine in Sport* 17(3): 261-265.
2. Burden, A.M. 2013. Abdominal and hip flexor muscle activity during 2 minutes of sit-ups and curl-ups. *Journal of Strength & Conditioning Research* 27 (8): 2119-2128.
3. Greene, M.E. et al. 2014. Diagnostic ultrasound imaging to measure the thickness of the transversus abdominis muscle during a supine abdominal bridge. *Journal of Athetlic Training* 49 (3 Suppl.): 5-101.

Curve Your Shoulders

1. Andersen, L.L. 2008. Muscle activation during selected strength exercises in women with chronic neck muscle pain. *Physical Therapy* 88 (6): 703-711.
2. Schoenfeld, B. 2011. The upright row: Implications for preventing subacromial impingement. *Strength and Conditioning Journal* 33 (5): 25.
3. Jerosch, J., et al. 1989. Sonographische befunde an schultergelenken von bodybuildern. *Deutsch Zeit Sportmedezin* 40(12): 437.

Develop a Pain-Free Upper Back

1. Jerosch, J., et al. 1989. Sonographische befunde an schultergelenken von bodybuildern. *Deutsch Zeit Sportmedezin* 40(12): 437.

Protect Your Lower Back

1. Fisher, J. 2013. A randomized trial to consider the effect of Romanian deadlift exercise on the development of lumbar extension strength. *Physical Therapy in Sport.* 14 (3): 139-145.

Enhance Your Chest

1. Welsch, E.A. 2005. Electromyographic activity of the pectoralis major and anterior deltoid muscles during three upper-body lifts. *Journal of Strength & Conditioning Research* 19 (2): 449-452.

About the Authors

Frédéric Delavier is a gifted artist with an exceptional knowledge of human anatomy. He studied morphology and anatomy for five years at the prestigious École des Beaux-Arts in Paris and studied dissection for three years at the Paris Faculté de Médecine.

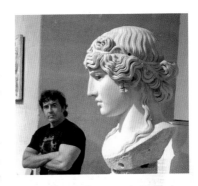

The former editor in chief of the French magazine *PowerMag*, Delavier wrote for several fitness publications, including the French magazine *Le Monde du Muscle, Men's Health Germany*, and *Ironman*. He is the author of the best-selling *Strength Training Anatomy, Women's Strength Training Anatomy, The Strength Training Anatomy Workout, Delavier's Core Training Anatomy*, and *Delavier's Stretching Anatomy*.

Delavier won the French powerlifting title in 1988 and gives worldwide presentations on the sport applications of biomechanics. His teaching efforts have earned him the Grand Prix de Techniques et de Pédagogie Sportive. Delavier lives in Paris, France.

Michael Gundill has written 13 books on strength training, sport nutrition, and health, including coauthoring *The Strength Training Anatomy Workout* and *The Strength Training Anatomy Workout II*. His books have been translated into multiple languages, and he has written over 500 articles for bodybuilding and fitness magazines worldwide, including *Iron Man* and *Dirty Dieting*. In 1998 he won the Article of the Year Award at the Fourth Academy of Bodybuilding Fitness & Sports Awards in California.

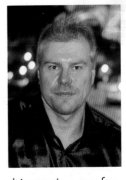

Gundill started weightlifting in 1983 in order to improve his rowing performance. Most of his training years were spent completing specific lifting programs in his home. As he gained muscle and refined his program, he began to learn more about physiology, anatomy, and biomechanics and started studying those subjects in medical journals. Since 1995 he has been writing about his discoveries in various bodybuilding and fitness magazines worldwide.

ANATOMY SERIES

Each book in the *Anatomy Series* provides detailed, full-color anatomical illustrations of the muscles in action and step-by-step instructions that detail perfect technique and form for each pose, exercise, movement, stretch, and stroke.

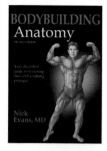
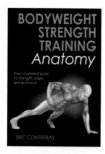
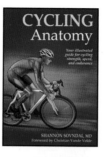
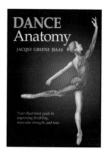
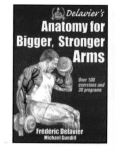

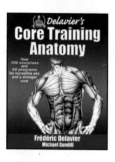
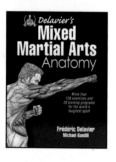
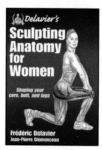
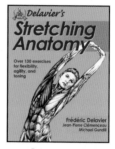
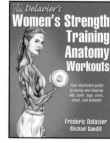

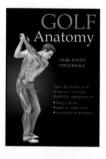
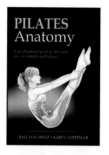
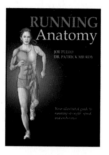
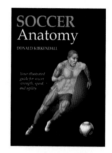
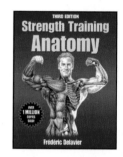

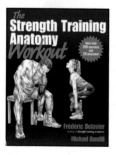
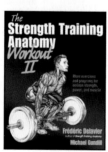
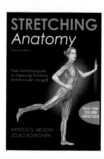
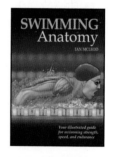
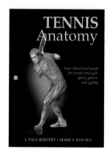

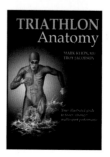
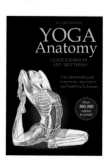

U.S. 1-800-747-4457
Australia .... (08) 8372 0999
Canada 1-800-465-7301
Europe .... +44 (0) 113 255 5665
New Zealand 0800 222 062

HUMAN KINETICS
The Premier Publisher for Sports & Fitness
P.O. Box 5076, Champaign, IL 61825-5076 USA